MAXIMIZING THE POTENTIAL OF YOUR OPHTHALMIC OFFICE

What You Need to Know About Planning and Design

MAXIMIZING THE POTENTIAL OF YOUR OPHTHALMIC OFFICE

What You Need to Know About Planning and Design

Fred L. Kahn
Design Consultant for optometry
and ophthalmology private practice offices

With a foreword by Irving Bennett, O.D.

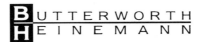

Boston Oxford Auckland Johannesburg Melbourne New Delhi

Library of Congress Cataloging-in-Publication Data
Kahn, Fred L.
    Maximizing the potential of your ophthalmic office : what you need to know about planning and design / Fred L. Kahn.
      p. cm.
    Includes index.
    ISBN 0-7506-7349-4
      1. Ophthalmology—Practice. 2. Medical offices—Design and construction. 3. Medical offices—Planning. I. Title.

RE72 .K34 2001
617.7'0068—dc21   2001035242

British Library Cataloguing-in-Publication Data
A catalogue record for this book is available from the British Library.

The publisher offers special discounts on bulk orders of this book.
For information, please contact:

    Manager of Special Sales
    Butterworth–Heinemann
    225 Wildwood Avenue
    Woburn, MA 01801-2041
    Tel: 781-904-2500
    Fax: 781-904-2620

For information on all Butterworth–Heinemann publications available, contact our World Wide Web home page at: http://www.bh.com

10 9 8 7 6 5 4 3 2 1

Printed in the United States of America

CONTENTS

ABOUT THE AUTHOR

In the mid-1800s, Fred L. Kahn's great-grandfather owned an optical supply firm that gave perhaps the first Canadian course in what became optometry. The course lasted one to two weeks, depending on how long a jeweler or druggist needed to learn the use of a trial set. The optical supply firm was eventually sold, and the author's grandfather and father started their own ophthalmic supply business.

Fred L. Kahn grew up on ophthalmic table talk and joined the family firm in 1946. Over the next few years, Kahn met some leading ophthalmologists and optometrists and was impressed by the struggle of Canadian optometry's leaders for recognition of their profession. The merit of their cause and underdog position appealed to him, which led to his office design activity.

Kahn told optometrists of his conviction that they will succeed best when their position as doctors is believable and respected. His message to them was and still is, "Your office (perceived mode of practice) must present the right evidence." In those days, recognition of optometrists as "doctors" was often damaged by the location of their office in the back rooms of a store. Then and now, better facilities encourage better perceptions from legislators, educators, and the public and help strengthen optometry's deserved status as a respected member of the health-care community.

Kahn's convictions were met with requests for help. Optometrists said, "Stop talking about it, and design a proper office for me." Being a civil engineer familiar with design drafting, Kahn started a sideline activity in office design for eye doctors and planned more than 100 private-practice optometry and some ophthalmology offices across Canada.

In 1968, Kahn met a gifted young designer/consultant, Larry Funston, whose first office design for an eye-care doctor revealed a rare mastery of his profession and a grasp of the images needed from and the services to be accommodated in a private-practice eye doctor's office. The author then devoted himself to and remains in "predesign consultation," the central theme of this book.

When the Kahn family supply business ended in 1981, Fred L. Kahn gladly accepted the invitation of Carl Zeiss Optical Inc. to offer design services full time. He is now semiretired from Zeiss, working from his home.

FOREWORD

Years ago Jack Runninger, then editor of *Optometric Management (OM)*, and I were on a cruise to Alaska with our wives. The two of us took a "busman's holiday" in Anchorage and, unannounced, stopped at a couple of optometric offices.

What a surprise to see on the desk of one optometrist a copy of the April 1974 issue of *OM*—the issue devoted in its entirety to the design for building and remodeling of a professional eye care office! The doctor told us that he had planned to build a new office and wanted all the help he could find. He noted that an office for an optometric practice needed to be somewhat "different." He had kept this particular issue for several years waiting for the building opportunity.

Fred Kahn, the author of the book you are about to read, is an expert in a field that begs for more experts. He has been there; he has done that. For the past quarter century that I have known Fred, I have come to appreciate his down-to-earth approach to office design; his meticulous concern with details; his imaginative and inventive ideas; and his budgetary concerns. I have admired his realism—no "head-in-the-clouds" person is he. And he's no "head-in-the-sand" person either.

Albert Fitch, the founder of the Pennsylvania College of Optometry, was one of the eye care profession's real pioneers. He is deservedly credited for numerous imaginative advancements for the emerging optometric profession. Fitch deplored advertising but he recognized the value of getting one's name before the public on a regular basis. It was he, then, who advocated that optometrists move their offices every five years or so and notify their patients and potential patients of the move.

Moving an office, erecting a new office, or remodeling an existing office can go far in building a successful practice or improving an established practice. This perception of progress in itself helps. An even greater help are the efficiencies that a new office can bring. In this day of managed care with its necessity to be more efficient (read that quicker), success is often predicated not only on doing a good job and but also in doing it in less time. This means, then, that an office that is not *planned* will often not provide the efficiency of patient and doctor movement. It will not result in the productiveness required with the use of ancillary personnel. And it will not offer the comfort of handling more than one task concurrently.

There is a quiet revolution taking place in eye care office designs. Form follows function and beauty follows both. Design is everywhere and the principles that govern fine architecture and efficient human engineering apply to eye care offices. The secret ingredients are imagination, a willingness to be innovative, and a desire to do a better job in delivering eye and vision care as never done before.

Not too long ago, I was driving from Philadelphia to New York with one of the principles of a firm for whom I was consulting. During the trip the gentleman said to me "Look up there on top of the very next hill. That's where I am building my new house." He proudly continued, "It is going to cost over a million!" "Why would you want to do that at your stage in life?" I inquired. He was in his 60s and his children were grown. "To make a statement," he exclaimed.

I thought a while and then blurted out "What exactly are you trying to say?"

If your office-to-be is a Taj Mahal and you have it built to exclaim to the world that you have made it, then I think this book is not really for you. The book concentrates on wholesome construction, intelligent floor planning, a "return on investment" venture that will provide a comfortable and convenient place to work and provide services with efficiency and effectiveness.

This book is unlike others published on this subject. It is a complete guidebook for the eye care world. It includes ideas that heretofore have not been considered by many eye care practitioners. The book will escort you through all the problems of fashioning and developing your outstanding workplace and offer you myriad possibilities on this journey.

You will enjoy the book. And you will benefit from reading it.

Irving Bennett, O.D.

PREFACE

The old adage is usually true: The best decisions are those made when you are best informed.

Maximizing the Potential of Your Ophthalmic Office: What You Need to Know about Planning and Design is an easy-to-follow guide for eye care professionals. You will learn the essentials of the complex and time-consuming process of relocating or renovating an existing office, or planning a startup.

This book includes many ideas for planning a facility. These ideas are wide ranging to meet many different situations, points of view, objectives, budgets, etc. Each doctor's career goals are individual to that doctor and his or her practice. In order to be successful, the planning processes and resulting designs must meet those individualities, objectives, and needs. Careful planning will ensure that office design will contribute generously to practice success and create the capacity to handle the necessary, realistically forecasted growth.

The book's inclusiveness and detailed planning processes have led to many checklists. These are organized to be easy to use and invite the description of this book as a "book of lists." You will learn to:

- List and prioritize your objectives (what this plan must do for you)
- Make a business plan for your own reference and to help get financing
- Know the expected timing for the investment to pay off

- Study the feasibility of the emerging project and promising alternatives to it
- Find a source of financing
- Decide whether to rent or own
- Choose a location
- Identify design criteria: all practice and other functions you want
- Plan for ways to respond to new and predictable changes in practice
- Know how office design can help you deal with competition, etc.

The book is organized both for read through and for reference on specific subjects. For example, feasibility ("Can it be done?"—and "Should it be done?") is addressed throughout the book, but the key area of "financial feasibility" is discussed at length in Chapter 13.

Patient and public perceptions of an eye-care facility make an underappreciated contribution to practice success. In this book, we will discuss how those doctors who are responding to a need, desire, or opportunity for a change in facility (usually a bigger, more impressive, and more effective office) will also benefit from a more positive public perception, which in turn contributes to the success of their practice.

Some of my past clients did far less planning than is outlined in this book, sometimes with no apparent damage to the execution or success of their project. You may prefer to be selective in your planning steps. However, this book will ensure that you are aware of most steps so you will know what you are omitting. It is even possible that as the planning and construction are underway, you will, perhaps at the last minute, decide to include some of the steps you left out. It is a bit ironic that a valid step in planning is to decide which steps to skip.

I hope that this book will be rewarding to eye doctors planning or considering a new office, and enjoyable to read. It also aims at being helpful and interesting to all others who have knowledge of or interest in these matters.

ACKNOWLEDGMENTS

Special thanks are due to Judy Cadle, both experienced and knowledgeable in the preparation of technical manuscripts for submission to publishers and in the operation and expansion of a big practice. She contributed knowledge, and then rare good sense in guiding me over the unfamiliar ground of writing this book.

Another special "thank you" goes to Dr. Irving Bennett, well known for his outstanding career as a practicing optometrist and unusual contributor to the building of his profession. He has given this book the benefit of timely and always to-the-point advice.

Sincere thanks to Charles Matthews, university professor and owner of a consulting operation in questionnaire applications and processing, for his role in producing the questionnaire answer report in the book.

Warm thanks to my adult sons, Peter and Stephen, for patiently teaching their "old" dad to use a computer in writing a book.

And finally, another warm "thank you" to the skilled computer input person, Susanna Graca, who converted my pages into a properly presented manuscript.

CHAPTER 1

First Steps in Considering and Planning a New Office

Be informed.

Decision Making

When you plan a renewed or startup ophthalmology or optometry office, including choosing whether to proceed, your decisions will be vital to your future. You'll want to be aware of and understand the many decisions you are likely to face, and how to judge opportunities and risks.

Start the process by gathering the kind of wide-ranging information available here and elsewhere. In all stages of such a venture, decisions based on appropriate information will optimize your chances and degree of success. Good decisions yield good planning, which is needed to ensure many things, including an office design that contributes generously to practice success and creates the capacity to handle the necessary, realistically forecasted growth.

Ideas, Checklists, "Read Through" or "Reference"

This book includes many ideas for planning a facility. They are wide ranging to meet each doctor's career goals and the many different situations, points of view, objectives, budgets, etc., that are individual to each and to his or her practice. The contribution of these ideas to the success of your planning and designs will depend on how well they meet your individualities, objectives and needs.

The book's inclusiveness and detailed planning processes have led to many checklists. These are organized to be easy to use. You will learn how and why to do the following:

- Judge the potential rewards and perils, and whether the rewards justify proceeding with the project
- List and prioritize your objectives (what this new facility must do for you)
- Make a business plan for your own reference and to help get financing
- Know the expected timing for the investment to pay off
- Study the feasibility of the emerging project and promising alternatives to it
- Find a source of financing
- Decide whether to rent or own
- Choose a location
- Identify design criteria: all practice and other functions you want
- Plan for ways to respond to new and predictable changes in practice
- Know how office design can help you deal with competition, etc.

The book is organized both to be read straight through and to be consulted as a reference on specific subjects. For example, feasibility (Can it be done? Should it be done?) is addressed throughout the book, but the key area of "financial feasibility" is discussed at length in Chapter 13. Patient and public perceptions of an eye-care facility that make an underappreciated contribution to practice success are discussed in Chapter 3.

An Existing Practice

In existing practices eye doctor/owners usually consider a major facility change in response to a recognized new situation such as a notable opportunity, a significant threat, a recognized need to update, etc.

If you are that eye doctor/owner, you will be making important decisions, such as whether a major change in your facility will be wise. The information needed for these early decisions includes:

- Identity and priority of your goals
- Identity and priority of things needed and wanted
- A business plan for that project in order to check the feasibility of your plan and of attractive alternatives, including financing the project being considered
- Advisability and factors involved in relocating
- How to choose a reliable way of proceeding with a move or expansion project
- The considerable range of things listed in this book's table of contents

Your high stake in selecting the best plan of action for this relatively unfamiliar venture will usually motivate you to search diligently for pertinent reliable information.

Even with excellent information, some of your decisions could be difficult. For example, do you proceed with a costly project if you encounter conflicting reports, one telling you that the patient share held by private practices is eroding (from patients going to alternative sources of eye care and eyewear), and the other telling you of growing strength in private practice patient share?

This is a real, not theoretical, possibility. I once encountered both at about the same time. Such conflicting stories would suggest that optimism or pessimism about private practice should be checked carefully, particularly in your area or region.

Practice Reaches or Nears Capacity: Choose and Plan Your Best Course of Action

Patient appointment delays are common and getting worse. Growth in patient numbers and practice income is stalling. Damage to the practice has become obvious. These and other things tell you that your practice is at, or closing in on, its capacity.

You want a continuation of practice and income growth. What are your options? Should or must you move? Can the present capacity be increased enough?

Visit other practices. Find qualified advisers, reputable management and marketing consultants who work with your profession, and ask them, "Without moving, how many more patients per day could we serve here with more and better utilization of staff, new equipment, better efficiency, etc.?" This should reveal the final capacity of your practice in your present office.

When you can see that your practice will reach final capacity within two to five years, start planning your next steps for dealing successfully with this problem/opportunity. Search for:

- Feasible and acceptable long-term alternatives to expansion or relocation
- The expansion or relocation project that will be best for you
- The right experienced advisors to work with you in your planning

Then, if the decision will involve a project, take the following action:

- Forecast growth in patient numbers and practice income after the project
- Make a business plan
- Find your financing
- Do the other things essential to making effective decisions about your project

Remember that your prime objective of return-on-investment (ROI, improved financial return from better income growth), should dominate any costly program/project for the solving of your capacity problem. What plan of action will be most likely to yield an acceptable ROI? What is the forecast amount of that feasible ROI?

At the time of the project, or when the need for one has been acknowledged, a strong practice-building program should be started, to help you get the fastest growth toward the needed ROI. Bear in mind that by its success, an effective practice-building program hastens your practice's next arrival at capacity. Therefore, if you are going to embark on a new facility project supported by a stronger practice-building program, plan for a large enough capacity to handle *accelerated* growth in patient numbers.

Choose reputable, suitable marketing consultants to guide this marketing program. Speed and magnitude of growth should justify the cost. Choose marketing techniques that match your personal ethics and your image as a doctor, giving primacy to your patients' best interests.

When to Start Your Planning

As soon as you can see that you will probably need a new office, start planning and forecasting for it.

You may deliberately or subconsciously postpone the start of planning, or ignore your capacity (or other) problems/opportunities, because the investment may exceed your comfort level. If you feel that there is no urgency, ask yourself, "How much advance time do I want for the kind of thorough planning I should do in this situation?"

A New Practice

As students, many doctors-to-be think (dream?) about becoming the owner of a truly successful practice. They often retain this ambition, even after gaining a good level of success in some other mode of practice.

If you are one of these, how can you judge whether your goals are probable, achievable realities, or just dreams?

- First, recognize that many dreams are the starting point for achievable goals.
- Second, do the hard work to inform yourself. Be a realist.

The realist says, "Show me." The realist wants contact with doctors who have been there. The realist wants *feasibility studies*, plus well-supported reasons why this is a worthy venture that should be expected to succeed. Optimists often say, "Go for it," which may invite unacceptable danger. Pessimists often say, "It sounds too risky," and may miss opportunities. The optimism of self-confidence is of course desirable, but realism in choosing your course of action is strongly recommended.

Check with Colleagues Who Have "Been There"

Colleagues who have completed a similar project are likely your best source of an objective story of the planning, implementation, and results involved. This is expanded in the chapters that follow and is presented at length in Chapter 14, "Colleague Questionnaire Report."

Phone as many colleagues as feasible and visit a few to see their facilities and their practices in operation.

This advice is so important it is promoted throughout this book. If you are uncomfortable about phoning an unknown colleague for advice, try working with prepared questions (see Chapter 14). The value of information from colleagues should motivate all but the most timid to develop a workable technique for doing it.

You may avoid making these calls because you have correctly told yourself that, "My community and/or circumstances are unlikely to be matched." You will have a point there, but similarities rather than close matching of communities and circumstances can be all you need. Some should be close enough for you to learn a lot, and get the reliable, experience-based information not otherwise available.

Try not to be deterred by the costs involved in checking with colleagues. These can include:

- Some travel
- Some time away from your practice
- Probably a much bigger long-distance phone bill

Where do you get lists of these practices? Consultants in practice marketing and management and designers of eye-care facilities have client lists and might direct you to some practices. Your state association might be able to help. Known colleagues, sales reps, and others with regional eye-care news (the grapevine) could also be good sources.

Feasibility Studies

For the existing practice, feasibility is covered at length in Chapter 13. For the startup practice, much of the business plan information in Chapter 13 will also apply, and there is a brief discussion of a business plan/feasibility study in Chapter 10 on startups.

Finding and Using Statistical Information

Use reliable statistical data in your planning. Your national association will be an excellent source.

Recent statistical data from the American Optometric Association indicate how infrequently an expansion or startup practice can be expected to lead smoothly to a strong, highly successful, eventually multidoctor operation. Despite that information, which I'm confident is reliable, you may want to consider the evidence of case histories of successful practices you contact whose stories establish that the unlikely *does* occur. This conflict emphasizes your challenges.

When you can get credible information about projects and can see that they are clearly successful against long odds, you'll see that effective planning toward your goals can lead to (though not ensure) success.

Self-Image

Your self-image can be a factor. It affects confidence, and confidence is often central to success. It can be pivotal in your decision whether to proceed with, postpone, or stay away from an expansion or startup project.

Does your self-image include *seeing* your practice:

- With expanded and improved clinical, dispensing, and management services?
- With you as a senior-executive style doctor in a multiple-doctor practice?
- Offering the widest range of today's expanding services?
- Using a well-developed program of management and marketing?
- In an impressive facility of 4,000 to 9,000 square feet?

Some eye doctors have a built-in self-image that says, "I will be very successful in my practice." Although that self-confident image is often in their genes, it can be developed and reinforced (or damaged) by experience. Try asking yourself "What kind of practice can I *really* create over the next five to ten years?" You may be tempted to answer, "I don't know" or, "It will depend on circumstances," and both would be valid. But an inner voice may speak more confidently.

Check the value of a strong self-image by that familiar method of calling on suitably experienced colleagues. You will easily recognize whether they have it.

Combine a confident self-image with knowing how to plan an outstanding practice, and you are much more likely to achieve it.

Professional Advisers: Who and When?

Once you decide that you need and want a better facility, plan to retain two advisers. Find both a top practice marketing and management person or firm, *and* a consultant/designer, each specialized in your profession's eye-care facilities. This team could be independent from each other (better?), or from the same operation. You retain them for their experience and knowledge, to provide you with vital planning assistance in identifying and developing ways of reaching your practice objectives, perhaps without a new facility. The cost of the two advisers should be acceptable when judged against the benefit they deliver.

For detailed information about the valuable things a suitably experienced ophthalmology and/or optometry marketing and management service can do for you, talk to the m/m service of your choice and see Chapter 11.

Neither the management/marketing consultant alone nor the design consultant is likely to know enough to advise you well enough in all of the important steps in planning your project, particularly if it is a big one. Many of those steps are listed below.

- Guide you through a "feasibility study" to evaluate your project and its alternatives, particularly from a management and marketing point of view

- Develop the necessary components of your business plan, pivotal for your planning, and for obtaining your financing
- Identify and weigh the advisability of less costly alternatives to a new facility
- Identify and help you weigh for prioritizing, the predesign factors that will control your venture, and the specialized facility planning you may need (these factors and planning are described at length in the chapters that follow)
- Direct you to colleagues who have completed similar or applicable projects
- Propose a marketing program and forecast its probable results
- Find the new practice capacity needed before another move will be required
- Advise on size of space and indicate benefits and drawbacks
- Help list and detail design criteria for all the practice functions (clinical, dispensing, administrative, etc.), in the new facility
- Provide reasonable guesstimates of cost
- Recommend location choice in general, and in particular among those available
- Prepare for the first preliminary, conceptual design of your facility
- Answer important questions from the vantage point of extensive experience

Your accountant will likely be needed for her/his knowledge of your practice numbers.

To avoid the cost and problems from duplication of services, decide early in the planning process the scope of each of your advisers' roles.

To find your two main professional advisers, get referrals from colleagues who have been there, and whose results you admire. Other leads for finding a designer/consultant can be to talk to an appropriate management/marketing firm; to find an m/m firm, talk to a reputable d/c. There are also the ophthalmic grapevine, a contractor you trust who is experienced in projects within your profession, a relative or friend with pertinent experience, etc.

Some doctors avoid using such advisers because of cost, and others because they're sure they can do it themselves—particularly if they recently took part in a construction project that greatly improved their know-how. But no matter how well you could do on your own, your advisory team's years of experience will almost guarantee that with their assistance you will do better (potentially much better). They are often needed when a project presents an unexpected critical problem:

- Questionable feasibility
- No obvious choice of location
- Overcoming at acceptable cost the flaws of an otherwise good location
- Needed items versus cost
- Landlord demands
- Technical problems such as land drainage or meeting local building codes

Start with professional advisers as soon as you decide to respond to the need, opportunity, threat, ambition, etc., you have identified, before putting a lot of your time into detailed planning. In terms of risk versus benefit, this will be good timing for a thorough examination of your objectives and alternatives, as well as your entire "workup" on your project to date.

They should make an early examination of your proposed strategies in response to the problems, opportunities, and/or ambitions that apply to your situation, such as:

- Your fast-approaching, or evident arrival at, practice capacity
- Need for a recognizably improved, up-to-date operation
- Space too small to accommodate new or expanding practice services
- No renewal available on your expiring lease
- Availability of a much better practice location
- Your decision that now is the time for you to start your own private practice

Your adviser(s) should discuss whether your project is likely to be the best way of achieving your objectives, solving your problems, taking advantage of your opportunities, and achieving your ambitions.

If they advise you to postpone or drop it, seriously consider doing so, but first ask for suggestions of alternatives. If they advise you to proceed and you agree, your adviser should suggest when detailed project planning should start.

Advisers' Fees

These vary. Weigh cost against the results colleagues have achieved using these or similar advisers. Most eye-care consultants (in design and/or management and marketing) who specialize in private practices will be flexible in their work scope and the related fees. You should of course be looking for a scope of work that will get the needed results, and a cost that is comfortable for you.

Omitting Planning Steps

Some of my past clients did far less planning than is outlined in this book, sometimes with no apparent damage to the execution or success of their project. You may prefer to be selective in your planning steps. If so, this book will let you know what steps you are omitting. You may decide to restore some of them. It is a bit ironic that a valid step in planning is deciding which steps to skip.

Healthy Doubts

It is obvious that you can achieve success in private practice without having a highly effective, impressive office that wins the right perceptions, even though such an office would almost always add greatly to the level of your success.

Some anecdotes will illustrate the point.

Two good friends of mine, optometrists, one in Canada and the other in the United States, both now retired, were both recognizably successful. The Canadian, whom I have known for many years, often went without lunch as an optometric student for lack of food or money. Having neither money nor credit, he opened a tiny big-city practice in two small rooms at the top of a long flight of stairs. His exam room was one thin partition away from a noisy radio repair shop. His practice soon outgrew his small waiting room, so patients sat on the stairs. Later, he gave up dispensing, installed his practice in larger but still modest space, still out of sight in an office building, and the practice continued to thrive, providing him with a fine income over many years. It became a three-doctor practice. During his career, he won recognition among his peers for leadership in continuing education and contact lens practice. Failing eyesight finally forced his retirement, unwanted because he enjoyed his practice so much and because so many patients kept asking for him, even phoning his home.

The American optometrist practiced in a small town with his brother, also in a modest-sized office, and his contribution to his profession and the ophthalmic field in general became well known throughout the United States.

Our family optometrist of many years, now retired, is of Japanese background. She ignored and overcame obstacles of race and gender that were oppressively evident in her early years, to have an inspiring career.

She started practice in the back of a small-town jewelry store. Though neither self-assured nor assertive, she had unshakably firm determination and winning charm. Her professional stature grew steadily as her outstanding work in children's developmental vision care won her unusual recognition and gratitude among her patients, their parents, and their teachers.

Although she had an above-average office, it played no more than a supporting role in her progress. Her story showed me many of the other factors that are central to practice success.

If you provide a service that the public values highly, word of mouth will build your practice, even if it is in a "hidden" location and you do no promotion (meeting with and talking to education directors, teachers, and parent groups, plus mailings, etc.). This certainly describes her situation, and yet she eventually had more patients than she could handle. A move to a new location, at a distance dangerous for most big-city optometrists, won't threaten a strong enough practice. She moved twice, once outside her patient area, and the other time to the edge of it. Each time, her practice improved its rate of growth.

Authoritative bad-mouthing won't hurt you if your patients appreciate you. A well-placed pediatric practitioner criticized her work to his patients. She didn't try to dissuade or refute him. She just kept helping kids, and her practice thrived.

A decor that identifies a racial origin and feminine gender can please and interest many patients. Subtle touches in her clever and appealing office decor paid tribute to her Japanese background and her femininity.

Even when you do nothing to promote yourself, it is possible to have a lot of militantly loyal patients, as illustrated by the following story. At our optometrist's invitation, my wife and I joined her at a lecture on children's developmental vision care, given at the Toronto Education Centre by an out-of-town optometrist who specialized in children with these problems. It was sponsored by and given to the parents in the regional Association for Children with Learning Disabilities. A small group of local optometrists also attended. The room was packed, mostly with very intent parents, as well as some teachers. After the talk, when the few optometrists present were chatting in the lobby, a group of ACLD members approached. They asked whether all present were optometrists (my wife and I stepped aside). Then, they firmly criticized them for leaving the essential care they were determined to get for their children to only one member of their profession, my embarrassed friend. Their children were her patients.

If you have been practicing for long, you will probably know similar stories, which quite correctly might inspire you. There is much to learn from such stories, particularly the dominant importance of being both an outstanding doctor and an excellent people person. But it is surely equally true that these doctors would have done even better in an appropriately effective and impressive facility.

My advice favoring top professional guidance remains firm, but must be qualified. With so much at stake, while having confidence in your professional consultants, you should continue to give clear and critical thought to all that you do, and listen to other reliable views. Apply healthy skepticism and careful thought to any career guidance you receive—including, of course, what you are reading here. Question what you are told. Say, "Show me!"

For example, experts who advise you that deep-pocket corporations will bury you with their contracts and marketing will be acknowledging the existence of such competition, but might be entirely wrong that you couldn't succeed. How else do you explain the success of optometrists and ophthalmologists who proceeded when conditions were as impossible as these predictions suggested?

On the other hand, if you're advised to proceed, you should still think about it. You might find some reasons why the venture won't be right *for you*, isn't timely, etc. Ask yourself, "Is there a better way for me to achieve my goals?"

Here are some examples that illustrate the general point about questioning accepted wisdom.

A school principal I know loved teaching chess to seventh and eighth graders "because they're old enough to learn the game." When his school became grades one through six, he continued teaching chess. Many youngsters did just fine. The accepted wisdom (his own) wasn't reliable.

Quite a few years ago, prescriptions for grade-school children were based on a working distance much longer than it actually is. One observant optometrist doubted the accepted standard and did some experimenting. A much shorter distance is now accepted.

As discussed elsewhere in this book, evidence doesn't sustain the widely accepted minimum population needed to support one successful optometrist. Practices are successful in these locations, despite the accepted lore. Clearly the doctors involved applied healthy skepticism to advice on population.

Even with the best advice, remain alert and well informed, as conditions can change. My optometrist friend of Japanese origin told me of putting her elderly little father, who spoke little English, on a Toronto-to-Montreal flight to visit another daughter. The flight's first scheduled stop was Ottawa. She repeatedly instructed him to get off at the *second* stop. After she left him, there was an on-board announcement, unknown to her, that the plane was going direct to Montreal. Her father vanished. Many hours later he was found in Rome, the next destination for that plane.

There is a very old story of a grandfather who put his beloved grandchild on a high wall, held out his arms, and said,

"Jump." As the little one jumped, the grandfather dropped his arms, letting the child fall to the ground. After picking up and comforting the crying child, the grandfather said, "Now don't forget. Don't never trust nobody!"

Skepticism is not a pleasant or easy route to follow. It flies in the face of the wisely and widely chosen practice of having confidence in the advice of experts with track records that you can (and should) check. You will be looking for your comfort zone in the middle ground between worthy experts and that traditional virtue of self-reliance.

Flow Chart: Early Steps in a Project's Planning and Implementation Processes

An overview at this point, covering approximately the first half of the book, is shown in Figure 1-1, which gives you a kind of map of the structure being explored. It is a flow chart of the early steps in a project's planning and implementation processes.

The steps named in this and later flow charts are of course expanded and discussed at length in the book, where the chapters and sections cover the flow chart subjects but are sometimes presented in a different sequence and with different headings.

For its limited purpose, a good flow chart should require little or no explanation. Being perhaps the most condensed and simplified way of describing a process, it offers two opposing effects: the advantage of quick exposure to the titles of the components, and the disadvantage that there are no details or discussion.

EARLY STEPS IN A PROJECT'S PLANNING AND IMPLEMENTING PROCESSES

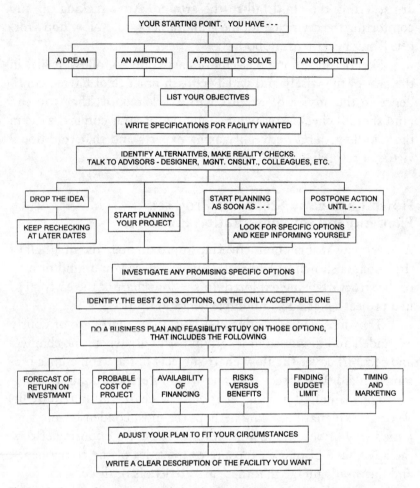

Figure 1–1   Early steps in a project's planning and implementation processes.

CHAPTER 2

Your Objectives, Your Design Criteria

Identify, Prioritize and Evaluate Your Objectives

Your next step in planning will be to identify, list, and prioritize your objectives, and then examine their advisability and feasibility.

Your **primary objectives** are your *big* targets, your most important goals, your best-considered reply to the question, "Why are you doing this?" They need to be described clearly and briefly, and should be more specific than "successful expansion" or "a successful startup."

These objectives and their priorities should and will control many of your project decisions (large and small), based on your answer to "How will this affect the achieving of my objectives?" By focusing on them, you will keep your project on track. For this to work, the list has to be as short as you can make it.

The objectives (goals) identified in many relocation and expansion projects often include some way of saying the following:

- Much better income
- Best response to the practice's problems and/or opportunities
- Faster growth from improved patient confidence
- Improved perceptions of my profession by the public, educators, and legislators

Return on Investment (ROI)

Although the targets just listed and others deserve their recognition, your top priority will often need to be *return on investment,* a bedrock reality. Without that return, you could fail to win your objectives and perhaps lose your investment.

I encountered this lesson in reality long ago, in a book titled *Editing the Day's News*. It opened with, "The first duty of a newspaper is to remain in existence. Otherwise it can't print anything."

This principle also applies to professional health-care services. Morally and legally, your primary duty is to your patients. But you can't provide any services unless your operation remains in existence, and you won't be satisfied unless it does a lot better than that.

Planning, designing, and contracting the expansion, relocation, or startup of your practice requires a serious investment. You must be confident of getting enough ROI to pay for that investment and yield a sound return

Your income increase is your ROI. It must be at least several percentage points better than you can get from a guaranteed investment. And both it and the project's payoff should be achieved in an acceptable time—perhaps five years (not including any real estate cost), although your accountant may advise longer.

Other Objectives

Although some objectives such as ROI are based on vital tangible dollar goals, others will often be nonmonetary.

After ROI, your objectives list may contain any of the three listed earlier, plus the following:

- Achieve my definition of success in my profession
- Respond effectively to my practice opportunities and/or problems
- Offer excellence in a full range of services
- Be recognized as a top health-care professional in my community
- Avoid or minimize the negative effects of "managed care" and other kinds of limiting contractual arrangements
- Enjoy my practice even more than I do now
- Attract my daughter, son, or some other worthy successor into my practice
- Have more personal time for my family and/or other interests

Other objectives could merit inclusion, but consider carefully since your list needs to be brief to be effective for its purpose of reference in decision-making about your project.

The Difference between Objectives and Design Criteria

"Objectives" are defined at the start of this chapter. "Design criteria" are descriptions of what will be needed for the accommodation of all services and functions in your reorganized and/or relocated practice, which starts with a list of those services, functions, etc.

To keep your list of objectives short, try to separate them from "design criteria." An example will illustrate. Quite often an eye doctor lists the important goal of greater efficiency of office layout as an objective, particularly when inefficiency is a daily irritant. But greater efficiency is more a means to an end (practice success) than an objective. Your objectives list will be shorter and your designer correctly guided when efficiency is a key item in your design criteria list.

Although essential practice service innovations are often listed as objectives, they and other frequently vital functional needs and wants are rarely a controlling reason for or primary goal of the project in the same way as return on investment. That is why they are usually listed as design criteria, not project objectives.

Additional design criteria might include the following:

- A clinical pod or at least two exam rooms per doctor
- A much bigger and/or greatly reorganized preexam operation
- A contact lens instruction/information operation using video and/or computer
- A private office per doctor
- Lens application stations and area
- A prescription lens production laboratory

Your list will probably be very different, and perhaps much longer. Your designer will need to know about changes to existing services and procedures, and the new ones to be added, to develop your design criteria for them. Remember, though, that most new exam-room functions (particularly those available through new technology) will rarely require more exam room space than is presently available or demand design changes there, as this would inhibit the vendor's sales of the product.

The design criteria for wanted and/or needed services and functions is a vital part of new eye-care facility planning. The criteria are presented in Chapters 5 through 10.

Developing your full list of design criteria for all needed services and functions will be a complex, demanding process. That is why you and your designer should use your combined experience in setting up your final design criteria lists. Make a complete list; then decide what to omit.

In choosing the inclusions and omissions in planning and designing your new operation, base your priorities on patient benefits and practice income. Balance those two advantages against cost for each item on your list.

Practice Capacity Controls Maximum Income Objective

Practice capacity is the maximum number of patients your practice can serve in a given time (day, week, month, or year).

In planning that involves capacity, use capacity per day, since it is easier for you and your staff to visualize. An accountant may use capacity per year for its influence on your annual practice income.

Plan for practice capacity large enough for your *final* income goals, not immediate revenue. That targeted maximum practice capacity will influence or control some important project decisions:

- The size of your new facility (for your eventual practice capacity)
- The cost of the space needed to permit the targeted capacity

Obviously, cost often influences capacity planning decisions. For example, despite higher cost, you may want more space now if your investigation suggests that a well-designed facility and well-organized operation will still not permit your practice to reach its targeted eventual maximum capacity well before you retire.

Consider a negative factor in this capacity planning. An American Optometric Association report, "Caring for the Eyes of America," compares population growth to the net increase in the number of optometrists entering the profession, and also notes the growth rate in patient visits to their optometrists. Both indicate that inadequate capacity will be rare.

On the other hand, anecdotal evidence tells us that many ophthalmology and optometry practices often operate at capacity. If your practice reached capacity once, it may happen again faster than before because of accelerated growth stimulated in part by the new office location, etc. Perhaps you should plan for that kind of growth. Before starting a project, decide which situation applies to you. Target a capacity that yields a good compromise between the cost of more space now, and the cost of moving later if and when the practice is again at capacity.

There is considerable spread in patients served per day in existing practices. In optometry, one doctor reported spending about five minutes with most patients and was closing in on his practice capacity. All "data gathering" was done by qualified assistants. Six to twelve patients were served per hour.

Other optometrists routinely book new patients for forty-five minutes and repeat patients for thirty. They, too, will reach numbers that threaten their capacity, but they could of course increase their capacity by finding acceptable ways of spending less time with each patient.

In the middle are the many optometrists who book appointments every fifteen to thirty minutes. Quite a few of these reach capacity, as revealed when they need to plan an expansion or some other project to let them serve more patients.

Similar variations in the average time the doctor spends with each patient occurs among ophthalmologists, although the time span and the factors affecting it will be individual to that profession, and the doctor.

Some practices experience slowed or stalled growth for reasons unrelated to capacity, indicating that other problems need attention. Be sure you really need a new office.

Before targeting the final patient *capacity* you want in your new facility, you will of course look at the eventual and "after five years" *income levels* feasible with that higher capacity operation. Information about feasible income per practice capacity should be available from:

- Qualified, appropriate management/marketing consultants
- Colleague friends (who may be understandably reluctant to reveal their income levels)
- Anecdotal information about colleagues
- Your national association's survey data
- Perhaps professional journals

Calculating Practice Capacity You Will Need in Your New Facility

Calculate your target for eventual annual practice capacity needed to earn the income you want, as follows:

1. *Find your present average billing per patient:* Divide your total annual income for the past year by the total number of patients (regardless of the services each patient received).
2. *Forecast your average billing per patient after the move:* Examine possible sources of new income, and get data from colleagues who made similar changes.
3. *Calculate the annual number of patients you must serve to reach your eventual income target:* Divide your income objective by the new average billing figure (item 2).
4. *Decide how many days per year your expanded practice will have a doctor serving patients:* The 1996 range was generally 230 to 270 days.
5. *Calculate average number of patients the practice must be able to serve daily, to reach the income target:* Divide the number of patients per year (item 3) by the number of "doctor-days" (item 4).

This is the daily capacity needed to reach your income target. To check the time this allows per patient, divide the total number of daily minutes that a doctor is on duty by the daily number of patients (item 5). If this is less time than is needed with each patient, then when that situation arrives, you will be forced to choose between reducing these minutes per patient or getting another doctor (perhaps part time). You will thus be deciding whether you should now take enough space for another doctor's pod ("pods" are explained later).

Forecast *when* you expect to reach this capacity. If it appears likely that you will need additional space for expansion relatively soon, and you can't get more space now, you may want to consider whether to proceed with the soon-to-be inadequate space project, accepting the prospect that you may face another expansion project sooner than seems economically wise, or look for bigger total space now. Some doctors welcome a further move as another "opportunity."

Practice Income at Capacity with Two or More Doctors

Although this is rarely central to your *early* financial results, you will often want to estimate the total practice income possible and whether it meets your target when you have additional doctors. (Remember that your personal income as doctor/owner is an entirely different matter that should, of course, be examined separately in your planning.)

Before calculating this maximum potential practice income, take the following steps:

- Forecast when another doctor will be needed, and when that doctor will be fully booked.
- Decide whether each doctor will have two or more examining rooms (perhaps in a pod) for most efficient use of the doctor's and the assistant's time.
- Decide the average time each doctor will spend with most patients.
- Decide how many exam periods should be reserved per day for the doctor to do non-patient-care things. Subtract these minutes from the total doctor-available time per day.
- Decide how many days per year doctors will be available to serve patients.

- Forecast the new, increased (?) billing per patient in the expanded practice.
- Calculate the total possible annual income when the practice is at capacity with two or three doctors, by multiplying (a) the number of doctors involved, times (b) the number of patients each doctor could see per day if fully booked, times (c) the number of days per year the doctors will be available, times (d) the new average billing per patient (averaged for the first five years).

Some Final Thoughts on Capacity

- Investigate whether the time needed to get enough additional gross and then net income for return on investment will yield a feasible project.
- See Chapter 14 for the answers to a survey questionnaire on results, some of which could help you with the suggested few colleague questions that follow.
- Ask colleagues if they have reached their capacity in their new facility, and if not, when they expect to.
- Ask these colleagues how long it took or will take for them to have the additional income to pay off the project.
- Get information on feasible income targets from your present practice and from authoritative survey data.

Once you know the income needed to justify each favorable version of your venture, it should be easier for you to recognize the most promising one. This personal decision will usually depend on your comfort with the goals you think are achievable, and the associated risks.

Investing versus Spending

Return on investment separates "investing" from "spending." This is a central distinction in considering and planning practice expansion, relocation, startup, or a related project. You will make the best cost decisions for your investment if you firmly focus on your probable prime objective of ROI.

Your parents probably gave you some wise advice: "Don't spend too freely, or you'll invite disaster." You *spend* when you buy a family car, a new outfit, a fine vacation, etc. You *invest* when you commit funds to make money. Before investing, you need reliable evidence that your investment will pay off, and how good that payoff (your ROI) will be.

The ROI from investing in the expansion and/or relocation of your practice comes from *additional* revenue. To merit the size of investment needed for a relocation or expansion project, the amount and rate of additional revenue must be well above normal growth.

Your decision to invest in this kind of project will therefore depend on answers to the following questions::

- How good is the evidence that enough extra revenue will indeed come?
- Where will that extra revenue come from?
- How much additional revenue can be expected?
- How quickly will the necessary additional practice revenue be earned?

Sources of Additional Revenue for Your Top Objective, ROI

You can hope to get additional revenue from the following sources:

- Higher billings per patient
- Additional patients served (new patients and more frequent eye care)
- Money saved from reduced costs

Let's take a close look at all three of these possible sources of additional practice income.

Higher Billings per Patient

On the clinical side, some major sources of higher billing per patient appropriate to a doctor are:

- Fees for new clinical services
- Increases in fees for existing but improved services

On the treatment side, in eyewear, more patients will want and therefore choose:

- Signature eyewear
- More fashionable, and in particular, more my-lifestyle eyewear
- Superior performance lenses
- Sun protection
- Sports, hobby, and industrial or on-the-job eyewear
- Accessories

In contact lens services, the improved convenience and performance of contact lenses, presented effectively and professionally, could lead to increases in billing per patient, and to increased numbers of patients wanting contacts or wanting to replace theirs with something better.

A higher average billing per patient will be difficult to forecast throughout the practice because you don't know the impact of an appropriately improved, and effectively marketed operation and its facility. Since, for optometrists, and dispensing ophthalmologists, the majority of the income increase will often come from dispensing, the person forecasting should if possible have experience with highly effective up-to-date eye-care treatment services, particularly eyewear dispensing.

Increases in average billing per patient have been reported to me that range from 15 percent to over 100 percent. Since this percentage will make a considerable difference to both the forecast and the reality of your new income (critical to your "business plan"), look for the advisor with the best track record.

You should be able to get good assistance in this forecasting from marketing/management firms specializing in your kind of practice.

Money Saved from Reduced Costs

With rare exceptions, most reports I've seen cite only modest savings, or sometimes none at all, from reduced costs. Explore this. Find your present cost per function. With your advisers, look for savings opportunities such as improvements in operational and management functions or a more efficient design. Again, check with suitably experienced colleagues. Even when the savings are modest, they can be worthwhile.

Additional Patients Served

In forecasting growth in patient numbers, consider whether you will have adequate capacity for it in your new facility. As noted earlier, to make this guesstimate, convert your present annual number of patients served (regardless of the service received) to the daily number (divide the annual patient total by the number of "doctor available" working days in the year). This simplified calculation will be accurate enough to permit most eye doctors and experienced staff to visualize the capacity of their present operation, and then judge the capacity needed for a larger, more efficient one.

The next question is, "Will enough additional patients come soon enough?" Evidence about this should be available from colleagues who've had a year (preferably several years) in their new office. I am often told that these numbers were above forecast, particularly in the first year, and still good after that.

Of the above three sources of additional revenue, "additional patients served" sometimes leads, but more often is a close second to, "additional revenue per patient." (See the report on the questionnaire answers in Chapter 14.)

Because this additional revenue is so critical to you, the following questions regarding "additional patients served" should be answered convincingly, to your satisfaction:

- What will cause the additional patients to come?
- How can I verify that they will come?
- In what numbers will they come?

What Will Cause the Additional Patients to Come?

What will bring enough additional people to you for eye care, and what patient benefit will influence the frequency of patient visits? In other words, *why* and *how often* will they come to you for eye care? Part of the answer is "perceptions" (discussed in Chapter 3), and another big one is the well-plowed land of practice building and marketing that offers many worthy ways of building patient volume in an established practice. A few of these are listed below:

- A more complete range of needed patient services
- More effective recalls
- Greater patient confidence in and comfort with the doctor and the staff
- Improved communication with patients
- Better-trained staff
- Public service and public relations activity
- Advertising

Now that you've examined the realities of your objectives and design criteria, inform yourself about the key support the success of your project can and should get from "perceptions," presented next.

CHAPTER 3

Perceptions, the Neglected Factor in Practice Success

Our Perception Is Our Reality

Perceptions are impressions sensed by observers. They are instant, subconscious responses to input that occur when someone or something has been noticed.

Perceptions are different from considered, deliberate thoughts. Although people usually have and can describe a perception about anything they encounter, they might have trouble answering the question "Why do you feel this way?" This is evidence that they are trying to describe a perception, not an analyzed series of thoughts.

Fortunately, perceptions are not carved in stone. Although first impressions tend to persist, further input can sometimes change them—for better or for worse.

Perceptions influence many of the public's choices of action— the personal day-to-day decisions to purchase this brand or item, from this source or that, or to vote for one candidate or another. Businesses serving the public, advertisers, politicians, and many others understand and use perceptions constantly. Perceptions thus have great importance in our lives.

For example, President Richard Nixon's five o'clock shadow tended to create a negative perception of him. Winston Churchill's jutting chin and direct gaze left a perception of courage and defiance. Adolf Hitler's body language gave the observer a perception of arrogance.

For many years, bank architecture consistently presented evidence of strength, solidity, and permanence. Courthouses are usually designed to provide a perception of dignity, unyielding standards, and dependability.

You will think of many more as you consider your perceptions of people and things.

Techniques for the selective presentation of evidence to influence people through their perceptions are becoming more varied and sophisticated as people become better educated and more aware, but the use of perceptions will continue to grow. If this worries you, bear in mind that any strong vehicle of communication can be used for both constructive and destructive purposes.

Using Perceptions to Build Practices

Perceptions are critical to the success of many ventures, including eye-care practices. They are discussed here to increase your awareness of this powerful force that can benefit your patients and your practice. The role of perceptions needs to be examined, understood, and effectively applied.

To attain your version of practice "success" in the shortest possible time, you and your practice must win the right perceptions in the minds of patients, strangers, educators, legislators, other health-care professionals, etc.

In eye-care practice, people's perceptions of an improved or relocated practice can strongly accelerate earnings. This has been so underappreciated that it merits the emphasis given here.

In ophthalmology and optometry, public perceptions of the facility can contribute powerfully to practice growth. Public and patient perceptions of you and your practice (affected in part by your facility) are also remarkably strong in attracting patients.

Your use of perceptions to build your practice faster after a move will depend on whether you are convinced they *can* do it. For this reason, the early part of this chapter briefly presented the results perceptions provide and why they work. Now, here is how you can use them.

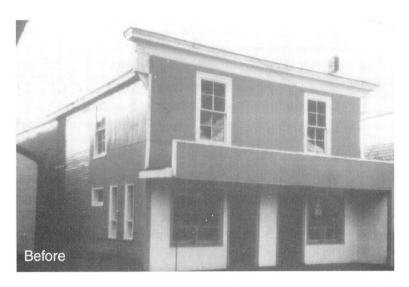

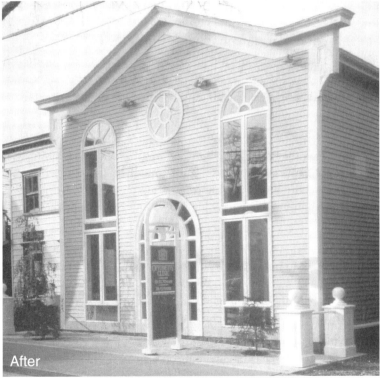

Figure 3–1 Don't dismiss an ugly duckling building as a possible location. It can become a head turner. This is a former store and fire station from the horse-drawn era bought and rebuilt for an optometry office. Its compelling appearance and historic interest will stimulate practice growth. (Reprinted with permission from Drs. Winslade and Pothier, Wolfville, Nova Scotia.)

Your office *exterior*, an often-overlooked marketing tool, should win public (nonpatient) perceptions of your practice that will attract new patients. Your office exterior should:

- Be visible and highly noticeable.
- Present the right evidence about you.

A well-known, respected jurist, when granting a retrial in appeals court, said, "Not only must justice be done. It must *appear* to be done." The same maxim applies to both the realities and the perceptions of you. Not only must you serve patients as well as they expect you to—you must also *appear* to be doing so.

A diploma on the wall isn't enough. For example, the evidence your patient encounters in your office (while under your professional care) may not support your doctor identity well enough. A patient or potential patient may see and/or hear things there that cause doubt about your doctor status, or about other attributes that patients expect of you and that build their confidence. If that happens (as it easily can), the patient may not return—there is no "retrial."

Ask a colleague who has been in a new office for more than a year (in your kind of population base) how much the patient and public perceptions of the new facility have helped the colleague's "practice growth" since the change. If you have made no effort to be sure that the exterior of your facility wins the right perceptions from nonpatients, you could be missing an important opportunity. This could be critical if you are facing serious damage from some third-party threat that is holding you back from a needed expansion project.

It is unfortunate when a successful, caring optometrist or ophthalmologist with high standards and a good practice has a facility whose exterior leaves nonpatients with a perception that does not match the reality of the doctor's excellence.

Doctors in that situation can be, and sometimes are, unusually successful. They do it by being so capable that they, their staff, and their practice reverse any perception of mediocrity. But their fine practice growth could be significantly greater if strangers who had no greater contact than seeing the office chose to become patients.

The Public Benefit from a Practice That Wins the Right Perceptions

An eye doctor's practice that wins the right perceptions is seen to be providing the high level of care suggested by the evidence. Its attractiveness (partly from its facility) will result in more people getting the benefit of its superior care.

Is Your Present Office Winning the Right Perceptions?

To be sure that you are getting positive perceptions from your present office, and/or to make the decisions about what you need in a new one, try to see it as a patient or stranger does. Turn a critical eye on the outside and inside. Ask yourself, "Do passers-by (driving and walking) notice my office? Does the outside give convincing evidence that will attract new patients? Does all that a person in my office sees and hears win the right perceptions?" Too often the honest answer will be "No," or "not well enough."

This can be hard for you and/or your staff to accept, since you have strong practice growth (referral based—the best way) and your office is so familiar and comfortable to you that you

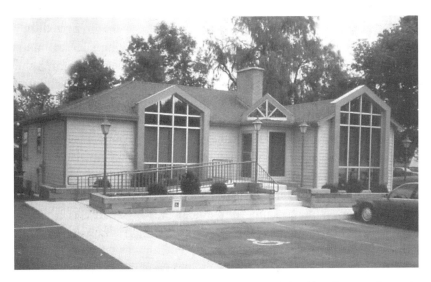

Figure 3–2 Satellite optometry practice in a plain-looking home adapted for its function and with a new, eye-catching appearance. (Reprinted with permission from Dr. James Day, Lamont, Illinois.)

have no reason to look at it critically. You may no longer see it as a visitor would, or really even notice it. (This blindness to the familiar is a common problem in marriages.)

Consider also the importance of perceptions that are potentially damaging with your loyal, established patients, when they encounter something negative at your office. You know that you and your staff are truly caring, competent people, in a patient-friendly office. Patients are happy. Why invest money to try for better perceptions? One valid answer is that these happy patients patronize other places (for nonoptical services and goods) that have been updated into improved, more attractive facilities that make them feel good, and more important—where they often feel catered to by the progress they see. When you don't make changes, your patient base could erode.

A facility that wins the right perceptions can help a practice be less vulnerable to competition, including the following interesting situation: Have you ever thought about the competition from all the merchants trying to attract your patients' consumer spending? Or why an eye doctor who is alone in a community still does much better with a strong, impressive facility? People in a one eye doctor town enjoy feeling that their doctor installed an outstanding operation *for them.* They think she/he really didn't have to, so they tend to feel proud that their small town has a first-class eye doctor. They come in more often, particularly the younger ones.

Another way to recognize how perceptions based on evidence attract or fail to attract patients is to consider your response to a poorly groomed sales rep. Consider a worst-case scenario (a caricature)—a person who is poorly dressed and sloppily groomed, who smells bad, has smoke-discolored teeth, bleary eyes, etc. This mess asks for your confidence. Your decision will come from your perception—the evidence, not words. You might even resent the feeling that the sales rep assumed you were gullible enough to trust him.

Credibility is the issue. You may know that your operation and staff are good, perhaps outstanding, and constantly improving. Is all the evidence of your facility, both outside and in, consistent with this reality of your excellence?

These perceptions are a key to practice growth and earnings. How important? Frankly, when I started this work (more than fifty years ago), I had no idea that the perception factor would be so important.

How do you verify this? Common sense (logic) supports it, but where is the evidence? Again, ask colleagues about their rate of growth after their change, and what parts of their new operation contributed the most. You will then have objective evidence for planning. Visit some of their offices and note your perceptions of them.

Integrity in Building Perceptions

Avoid false impressions that can come from unintended or, far worse, deliberately misleading evidence. Most of us encounter this far too often and usually dislike it intensely.

I was once challenged by someone who said that talking about perceptions was advocating flim-flamming. My critic felt I was urging unethical action—to make people believe untrue things. He cited the constant bombardment of media evidence to win public perceptions that will influence us to buy, vote, and support things that are less than or totally not what the evidence claims or suggests.

The public is indeed exposed to misleading evidence and is becoming increasingly wary, and even hostile when their expectations aren't met. But this also increases their appreciation of integrity. You already know that integrity tends to win strong patient support and loyalty.

You also know how immoral (and often ineffective over the long run) it is to try to win perceptions that are false, although we all have seen this done in the selling of products, politicians, and ideas. Your decision on integrity will depend on your personal ethics, perhaps influenced by your observation that truthful promotion, done well, can be powerful and much less vulnerable to attack.

The next vital question is, "What perceptions do you want people (patients and nonpatients) to have of you?" Your answers are your perceptual targets.

Key Perceptions That Produce the Fastest Growth

Among the many public/patient perceptions important to the growth rate of, and patient confidence in your practice, four seem to be leaders. You and your practice should always be instantly, undeniably perceived as:

- Truly successful
- A doctor, not a merchant
- A doctor of unyielding high standards
- A doctor (and a practice) with excellent good taste

Be Perceived as Successful

Most people want the confidence and sense of self-worth they get from perceiving that they are going to a doctor who is "excellent, one of the best, a success."

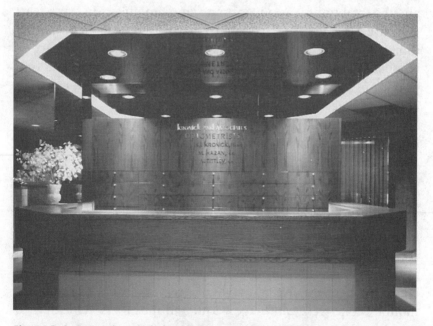

Figure 3–3 Reception and checkout counter at the entrance of an upstairs, small-town practice, designed to be impressive, suggesting success, high standards, and good taste. (Reprinted with permission from Drs. Joseph Kronick and Morris Hazan, Hawkesbury, Ontario.)

Some doctors are uneasy about being perceived as a success. They ask, "Won't I lose some patients who feel I will cost too much?" In my experience, some practices will indeed lose a few, usually those patients who are looking for the lowest cost and biggest discount.

Marketing experts oppose the policy of trying to be seen as all things to all people. In a mixed-income community, doctors who offer low fees and discounts may attract people who base their choice of eye doctor on cost. But they will damage their credibility with those (the majority?) who want to be sure they are entrusting their care to someone they perceive as a first-class doctor.

Even in communities where almost all people have lower incomes, patients usually want to receive fine care, even though they will often regretfully accept less on the dispensing side. People at all economic levels want to feel that first-class care is available to them, regardless of where they live, or the demographic profile of their area.

Don't fall into the trap of basing the policies (marketing and others) of your practice on exceptional situations. This could hurt your practice seriously. For example, you might decide to offer discounts or promote low prices because a small but vocal number of patients criticize your charges. This is a parallel to a common and useful old saying in teaching lawyers, "Hard cases make bad law."

Be perceived as truly successful to gain the many while losing the few (the "hard cases that make bad law" in your practice). Although this guideline is appealingly obvious, it is often ignored in policy setting and in doctors' responses to what may be only relatively minor problems.

Be Perceived Instantly and Incontrovertibly as a Doctor

Ask yourself, "Would I send someone I love to any doctor if I felt the doctor's decisions might be based on his or her wallet (making money), rather than on the best interests of the patient?"

Be instantly and with certainty recognized as a *real* doctor. It will give you great competitive strength, often vital to your success in the eye-care picture of today and tomorrow. Further, you, your practice, and your profession have much to gain in the crucial area of public perceptions when legislators, educators, and other people perceive you convincingly as what you are: a respected health-care professional—a doctor, not a merchant.

In general, the public expects a doctor to put patient welfare first, a different point of view than is commonly expected among merchants. I have no quarrel with merchants, many of whose ethics deserve a full measure of esteem—a merchant can be as ethical as a doctor, or more so. But a merchant's assumed priority is the sale, and customers expect to take some responsibility for themselves.

How do you present valid and convincing evidence that you are a doctor, not a merchant, while you offer a highly superior eyewear operation? We'll deal with this important challenge later (Chapter 7).

Be Perceived as a Doctor of Unyielding High Standards

The credibility of your image is at stake. Only when you present consistent and complete evidence of your high standards will patients have the conviction that you are as good as you really are.

Be sure, of course, that you indeed have unyielding standards. You may want to evaluate all that is done, said, and seen in your practice, and then make any necessary changes. As you make this important evaluation, remember that *all* evidence must support the perception of the high standards you insist on throughout your practice.

One owner proudly showed me his new location, a building renewed both inside and out. Meeting me outside, he asked, "Well, what do you think?" I had to tell him, "The building looks great, but how can you live with a lawn that's mostly mud and weeds?" He angrily pointed out that he hadn't discovered oil or gold on his property, and the lawn would have to wait until he could afford it. Do you agree? Or was this evidence that he could live with something substandard and damaging to him—so damaging that he should have found the money somehow?

Your need for evidence of excellence throughout your operation introduces the valid, important subject of cost. Often an eye doctor needs to concentrate on cutting costs to control or reduce the size of her/his investment. Such cost cutting should be chosen

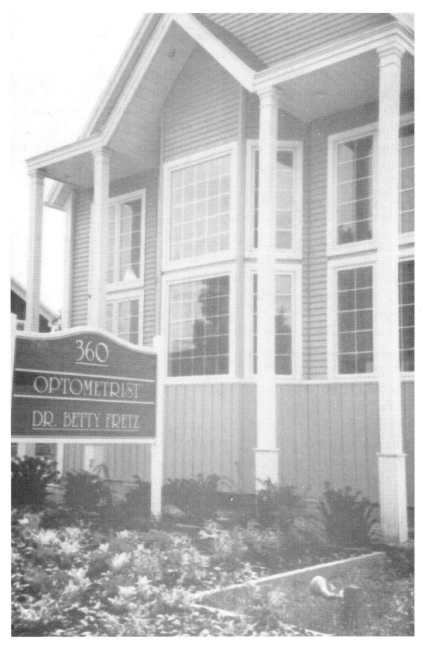

Figure 3–4 Former church, redesigned for optometry practice, illustrates the doctor's distinctive standards and should be recognized by the residents as a compliment to them. (Reprinted with permission from **Dr. Betty Fretz, Listowel, Ontario.**)

with the greatest of care. Your level of future success may be at stake. You are investing, not spending. With an investment, your objectives must be met—especially your need for enough income to pay the costs and leave you a good return. Your feasibility study should set a firm budget limit, within which you judge each proposal's cost against its affect on your ROI. Budget cuts need to be chosen so you avoid omissions or delays that leave evidence that you *don't* have unyielding high standards—that you can live with mediocrity and mess.

You, Your Staff and Facility Must Be Perceived as Having Excellent Taste

You dispense eyewear. To most patients eyewear means unwelcome changes in their facial appearance. Those short sentences explain why the general populace has suffered for many years from their reluctance to have the eye care from which they would benefit. They lose necessary health care and other important help because they don't want to wear glasses. Most people still resist wearing glasses (some strongly), despite great progress in many aspects of current eyewear fashion and its marketing. Dislike for wearing glasses is behind most refractive surgery and the success of contact lenses.

Outside the ophthalmic field, the cosmetics industry's wealth is based on public sensitivity about facial appearance. Despite new interest in eyewear (such as signature styles), the rejection of eye care based on that dislike remains strong, negatively affecting eye-care practices.

Consider the acceptance of contact lenses. Many early eye doctors would surely have laughed at the idea of the public demanding the right to put a foreign body on the eye, with no guarantee of success, at (then) relatively high cost, and despite the frequent physiological and psychological mechanisms of rejection. Yet the widespread dislike of glasses is so strong that the contact lens professions and industry are successful.

Today, more and more people are asking, sometimes impatiently, for expensive and somewhat risky surgery on their healthy eyes—not in response to pain or threatening illness, but because they dislike wearing glasses.

The power of people's sensitivity about their appearance in glasses seems so totally persuasive that it is hard to understand why it is treated so unimaginatively, casually, and even poorly in the eyewear operations of so many eye-care practices.

Does your practice, and especially your eyewear area, present reassuring evidence of a pleasing eyewear experience, leading to a happy result? Positive patient perceptions, based in part on evidence of good taste throughout your practice, will improve the confidence and positive attitude of those selecting eyewear, and their referrals will attract more patients. (See Chapters 7 and 14.)

Other perceptual targets could merit inclusion, but top priority goes to the preceding four.

Patients and others, after encountering your practice facility (outside, as well as in), will have responses and perceptions, often deeply felt but undefined, which can be positive, neutral, mixed, or even negative. In the instant needed to form perceptions, the right ones must occur and triumph.

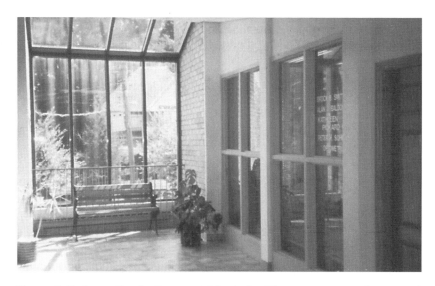

Figure 3–5 Appealing hallway outside their office entrance on the second floor of a health-care building suggests the excellence of their location and their practice. (Reprinted with permission from Drs. Kathleen Pickard and Peter Sohier, Simcoe, Ontario.)

Do you need proof of these benefits from the right perceptions? Once again, ask your colleagues. Those with new offices will usually tell you about their experiences and their results. These points were addressed in a client questionnaire, the answers to which are presented in Chapter 14. Ask your colleagues:

- "Was your move successful?" Among other things was/is ROI satisfactory"?
- "How many years did or will the project take to pay for itself and yield a fine ROI?"
- "Do you think 'perceptions' of your practice helped build patient confidence?"
- "What would you do differently if you were starting your project now?"
- "Has it improved your status with the public and other health-care professionals?"
- "What advice do you have for me?"

This chapter has offered you a general understanding of the role of perceptions in your venture's success. With that in the back of your mind for decision-making, it is time to look at specific choices you will be facing, such as your location.

CHAPTER 4

A New, Larger Facility

Choosing Your New Location

The old saying (approximately) that "the three most important things for success in serving the public are location, location, and location" seems to have merit. Location will be highly important in getting you the results you need from your facility.

Your list of what will make a location feasible and strong for *your* practice will probably contain many points identical with those of most others in your profession. But priorities for these points probably will vary a lot, depending on individual circumstances.

Factors in Choosing a Location

You should decide how important each of the following location factors is to you.

Visibility (Essential for Noticeability)

Visibility permits passersby to see your office exterior and thus have perceptions that should of course be designed to attract them. Your facility must be perceived as distinguished, both for itself and compared to other nearby buildings. Well-used visibility and noticeability speeds growth, even for well-established practices.

A visible free-standing building has excellent potential for yielding superior perceptions. When the office is in a well-known, respected health-care center or other fine office building where practice visibility is absent, you will have to rely on the public perceptions of the building, its address, etc., to win the desired perceptions.

Traffic Passing

Obviously the number of people passing your location on foot or in cars is critical to the benefit you can get from even the best visibility/noticeability.

The high volume of pedestrian traffic in busy shopping centers ensures excellent exposure, but there is a down side. A shopping center location can give incorrect or mixed perceptions of you (doctor versus merchant), unless your front design so convincingly identifies you as a doctor that it overcomes the expectation that in this location you must be a merchant. See the later section, "Should You be in a Shopping Center?"

Car traffic can be as effective as pedestrian if enough drivers and passengers notice your building and signs, and if that building and those signs win strong perceptions that you are a doctor, successful, etc. Visibility to fast-moving highway traffic can be valuable, but slower traffic on a busy artery with traffic lights can be better. Visibility from both, with access off the artery, will be better again.

In smaller communities (usually a town, not a city), the location of a new operation or the relocation of an established one

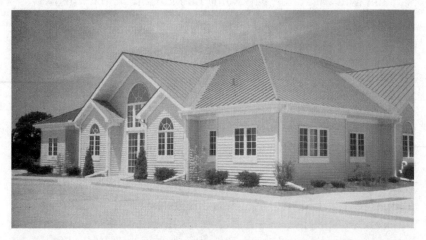

Figure 4–1   New, eye-catching, impressive free-standing building on generous grounds, designed for eye doctors' practice. A fine example of an investment justified by the rate of practice growth and many other benefits. (Reprinted with permission from Drs. Dale Kaney and Todd Bussian, Freeport, Illinois.)

becomes quickly known by word-of-mouth. At the same time, a startup practice there that is visible on a main street will usually need the good marketing benefits it will get from passing traffic. An established small-town practice would benefit from but not need the passing traffic if it moves to a building that is conveniently located and appropriately impressive.

Perceptions of Your Practice

Where feasible, choose or erect a building in an attractive neighborhood, or at least in a location within a chosen area that has no incompatible buildings or other unfavorable distractions. Negative evidence could cancel the benefits of even a distinguished, free-standing building that would otherwise do a fine job of winning perceptions that you are a successful doctor with unyielding high standards and excellent taste.

Other kinds of locations, such as storefront space on an appropriate street, can work well if the exterior appearance shows clearly that you are a doctor, distinctive, and excellent.

Parking

Parking is almost always a big factor, because convenience influences the "where-to-get-it" choices of so many people—although perhaps less often with health care.

Downtown practices in cities or large towns usually receive plenty of complaints about the difficulty and cost of parking. Why do shopping centers have trouble keeping handicapped parking spaces for those who need them? How often have you been frustrated driving around a parking lot, or a block, watching for someone to leave a space? How often have you complained or heard a complaint about "paying a fortune" for parking? How often do you choose a store or service for its convenient, no-cost parking?

With a new building, parking space numbers should be planned carefully. Local regulations usually dictate minimum parking spaces per building size. Since your aim is patient convenience and ease, the legal minimum will usually be too small—if not now, then in the future. Plan for generous patient and staff parking, to allow for strong practice growth.

Cost

Here's the factor that often changes doctors' location practice priorities. Concern about cost is of course wise, but strong anxiety can bring one or more of the following future problems that could be worse than budget pressure:

- A facility too small for your future space needs
- Omission of a pod per doctor, or of at least two exam rooms each
- No space to accommodate an additional doctor
- An inadequate business office
- Failure to improve an unattractive or undistinguished building exterior

Too often doctors tell me they later regretted that cost led them to scale back a design in a way that eventually had a serious negative impact on the practice. On the other hand (much less often), I have been told by doctors of their regret at failing to hold down costs, which led, for example, to financing difficulties.

Deal with cost carefully. If you choose the location with the lowest rent or the lowest installation cost (appealing ideas), it could be more costly in unrealized income.

Find an excellent location first, and then look for the least damaging ways of holding down costs. This is usually done best by you, your designer, your management consultant, and your contractor, working as a team and applying their respective experience-based knowledge.

Cost control needs a feasibility study that weighs the investment needed to achieve your objectives against the forecasted and necessary new level of practice earnings.

Financing

The availability of financing can control location feasibility. Before talking to possible lenders, you and your financial advisers (practice management consultant and/or accountant) should set your budget limit from income forecasts you have done together and checked for reality with appropriately experienced colleagues, as described in Chapter 13. Your budget limit is the project cost that must not be exceeded—a key part of your business plan that's essential for both your guidance and your loan application.

Your designer and/or general contractor, if experienced enough with eye doctors' projects, should be able to give you cost estimates (usually bracketed between higher and lower dollar figures) for those project locations that seem likely to be near your budget.

The project cost will of course have to be held within the financing available. If you need more money for the legitimate reason that the return will justify it, try to persuade your lender. For your present lender or a new one to have the confidence to improve your financing, he or she must agree that a location involving somewhat higher cost will generate a much better return. Unless enough money is available at acceptable rates for installing your practice (usually called "leasehold improvements") in an acceptable location, you may have to reduce your project to the lender's limit. If that will be seriously damaging, you may have to postpone it. For this kind of venture, the importance of your lender's confidence in you and your preferred location merits the guidance of experts in bank decision-making. (See Chapter 13.)

Population of the Area

The published figures I have seen for minimum population to support one private-practice optometrist seem seriously inaccurate. I have been told, and disagree, that these unreliable figures at least give you a benchmark from which to work. This topic has already been discussed in the section "Healthy Doubts" at the end of Chapter 1.

Here are two more bits of evidence. An optometrist successfully invested $500,000 in a new facility in a town of only 1,500. Another, in a town of 4,000, invested more than $600,000 and reports remarkable results. In these examples of a "too-small" population base, success seems based on superior doctors, using an effective marketing program, practicing in a strong, impressive facility.

Anticipated Changes in the Area

Sometimes demographic changes in your targeted area are foreseeable. A factory may be opening or closing, affecting local job opportunities. New subdivisions may be coming. Population may be dropping because of a bad economy.

Find out at the local municipal office (Chamber of Commerce) what developments are underway or anticipated. In smaller places, ask the local newspaper what is known or is rumored to be happening in the local economy. Find out from bankers and real estate agents about population changes and their causes. Check these reports with others to compensate for possible biases of civic pride or vested interest.

Note carefully any interest in attracting you to the area, or in helping you in some way. List the names of all the people who encourage you to come.

This last point is a valuable idea. Your investigation is a great way of developing a rewarding group of strong supporters, who will have an active interest in your success because they believe that you located there as a direct result of their advice. You could be shy about starting conversations with strangers who don't know you as a doctor—and doing it on their ground, rather than in your office. However, these conversations can be so valuable that you should try to schedule them, perhaps for a matter of hours per week for quite a few weeks. This idea is detailed in Chapter 10, "Planning an Office for a Startup Practice," but is equally valuable when you are investigating a move out of the market area where you are known (such as could occur after a massive ethnic change to a language you are unlikely to master—which has happened).

Investigate so you will know what to expect in your targeted community, neighborhood, or area. With thorough location research, surprises should be rare.

Timing in the Life of Your Practice

If this is a startup practice, your priorities on these points about location choice will reflect it. (See Chapter 10.)

Do you expect to be there for the rest of your practice life? Depending on your age and goals, this new location may be just right for the balance of your career, although it could hinder the sale of your practice a little if your prospective successor sees a need to move.

Based on their forecasts, some eye doctors expect their project to accommodate all future practice growth. However, strong moves supported by good practice marketing programs tend to produce growth above forecast. This might justify trying for more space now.

How Much Space?

Use the experience of qualified advisors to target a tentative office size based on functions and earnings. Then, start a thorough investigation of the feasibility and wisdom of that target.

This can be a difficult decision. Logic and prudence suggest, "Hold down cost—keep it small," but that could bring capacity problems far too soon. You may change your mind several times and still feel uncertain. You want a facility big enough for all your practice functions and financial goals for a lot of years. But space costs money. You will be judging cost versus benefit. Up to a certain size, there will be compensating benefits, but at what size will the benefits stop paying off?

Some doctors have a positive basis for a cautious approach to acquiring space. They view a subsequent need for another move with its further costs, etc., as a normal, entirely acceptable part of their career path. Since each project must be justified by its return-on-investment, they see a future move as another opportunity to improve their incomes even further through another period of accelerated growth, stimulated by the impact of their next, even more impressive, improved facility.

Both of those answers about facility size can be sound. Choosing the right size for your situation and your forecasted prospects won't be easy. Again, ask colleagues who made this kind of move, "Are you satisfied with your choice of size?" You may be reassured to know that in a survey I made of optometrists with project experience (see Chapter 14), less than half of them would have taken more space. Choose the approach and size that make you comfortable.

The designs presented in this book show what was done in different office sizes. The personal and fixed individuality of each of these doctor's situations cannot be presented (confidentiality), so you will be seeing the results of compromises for which the reasons other than space size will be unknown.

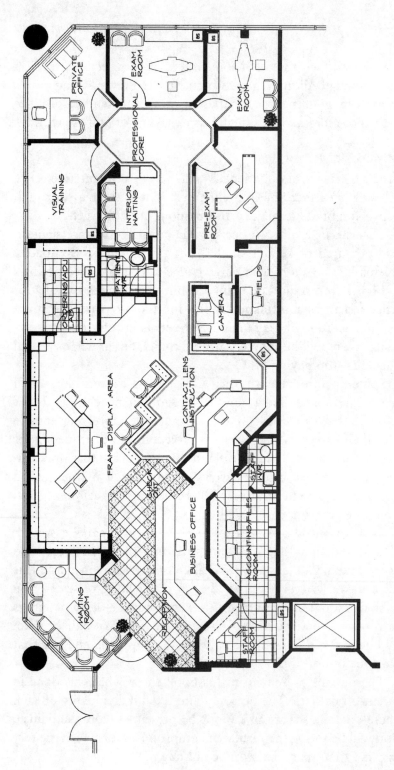

Figure 4–2 Plan of relocated, established, somewhat specialized practice in ground-floor space of a professional building. Plan based on her views, the shape of the space, its windows, and its building (2450 sq. ft.). (Reprinted with permission from Dr. Terry Ellen Noel, Allentown, Pennsylvania, population 105,000.)

These plans, presented here and in Chapter 11, are there through the generous consent of the doctor/owners, which included allowing me to use the practice name, location (community), and area, with a very brief comment on the project. The range of these example plans has one potential limitation: they are all the work of one designer, my associate Larry Funston, whose firm, Oadbe Associates, also gave permission for them to be shown.

If you want to see other plans before you proceed, your designer of choice may be willing to send you a portfolio of designs (with some covering explanations) chosen because the conditions come close to matching yours.

How Far Can You Move Safely?

For a relatively new practice, stay as close to your present location as you can, within sight of it if possible (the cautious approach).

An established practice can safely move to a strong enough location a mile or more away. Obviously an equally strong, nearby location would be better, but proximity to the previous place will rarely mean much if the new location is well marketed and markets itself well.

Should You Be in a Shopping Center?

The advantage of a mall's shopping concourse level is its high volume of pedestrian traffic (the basis of its higher rent). There are at least three possible scenarios for an eye doctor's office located on a mall concourse level.

- Eye-care practices have almost always been a destination, rarely a drop-in place. Doctors work to appointments often booked well in advance. Most people in a mall expect immediate mall-type service and would be unhappy at the delay (usually a matter of days).
- Some people in malls don't expect immediate service and could happily make a future appointment while enjoying the convenience of a shopping concourse location.
- A growing alternative is a shopping-level practice that serves most people immediately or after only a short (less than an

hour) wait, as in the growing number of medical drop-in centers.

Even on the professional offices floor, shopping center conveniences can be valuable. And for fastest growth to the highest gross income, a concourse level location in a shopping center sounds promising. There you are likely to meet your growth and income objectives quickly.

However, when a powerful, deep-pocketed, strongly promotional competitor turns up, as is very likely in a big mall, you will probably be seriously hurt. Even your attractive and noticeable front (distinctively that of a doctor, not a merchant) will rarely have the stopping power of the promotion-minded optical outlet and/or discounter nearby. Your location will then no longer receive the shopping concourse benefits that you pay for in your rent.

An ophthalmologist chose to have an office on the shopping level of a large suburban mall. It has an appealing but professional-looking front appropriate for a doctor. His immediate results look good. The long-term results remain to be seen. If your self and targeted image is "a recognizable *real* doctor," you will probably be uncomfortable located on a shopping-mall concourse level, because your location will send mixed signals to passersby: are you a doctor or a merchant?

Your doctor identity is a great strength for you in these challenging times, because many people want to be sure they are entrusting all parts of their health care to "real" doctors. That identity should be established and constantly supported by consistent, noticeable, fully convincing evidence, to give you the strength you need to compete with high-profile, promotional, deep-pocket operations. That point seems authenticated by the success (despite tough competition) of eye doctors with firmly established doctor identity—who, incidentally, rarely seem to be located on mall shopping levels.

So, your choice of a shopping center location will depend on your goals and what you see as effective and acceptable methods of achieving them. Time will reveal your wisdom or folly.

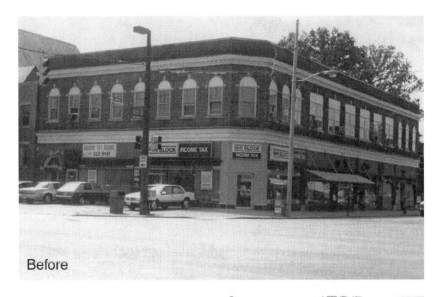

Before

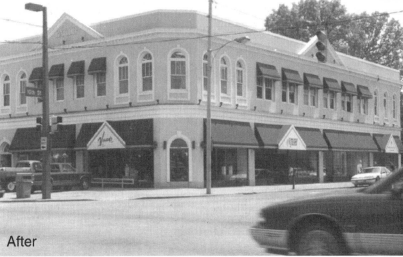

After

Figure 4–3   The doctors, practicing successfully in modest space in this plain downtown building, needed to expand and do even better. They bought the building, remodeled it to win strong, positive perceptions, and took almost all of the ground floor. (Reprinted with permission from Drs. William and Chris Ratcliff, Huntington, West Virginia.)

Should You Be on a Main or Side Street?

This choice will be influenced by:

- Your self-image
- Visibility
- Cost versus earnings
- The size of the community
- Whether your practice is a startup, in its early days, or established

In a big community such as a city, the choice of main or side street for an established practice could depend on its present location and thus where its patients would expect it to be, your patient base demographics, and the availability of appropriate space.

In a city location, find or create advantages consistent with your goals and desired image—perhaps an admired, well-known building with excellent parking, on a familiar street. Your notice-ability will have to be cleverly contrived to stand out in the great

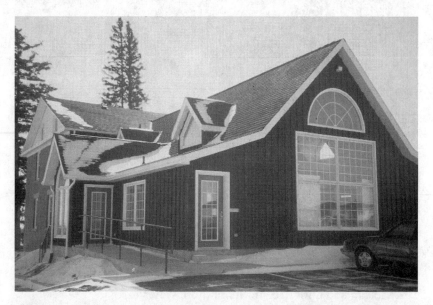

Figure 4–4   This well-known building, and their tastefully installed health-care use of it in the back addition, gave this practice (relocated from a shopping plaza) a stronger identity. A great location if you can find one. (Reprinted with permission from Dr. Stephen Code, Kitchener, Ontario.)

clamor for public attention—signs, building exteriors, exterior lighting, etc.

One doctor in a small city found an old home that was being considered for designation as an historic building. With an unchanged front, and the necessary addition in back, the city accepted its use as an eye-care office. He had a well-known location and local gratitude for conserving the appearance and character of the building, while using it for community benefit.

Another doctor won city approval by moving an old home to a new location. This cleared his old lot and saved its tree, which was appreciated in the neighborhood.

In smaller places, an established practice on a side street will be helped by a strong, noticeable exterior that wins the right perceptions, as with a notable free-standing building. This can contribute more to success than a much less attractive place on a main street.

An early-days or startup practice doesn't yet have the community awareness and recognition of an established practice. It needs a location that can win rapid public knowledge of its presence. An attractive and visible building with good parking on a main street can speed up its growth, but because circumstances vary, there is no formula.

Most practices, but particularly a startup, will gain from being in a well-known building or close to a local landmark—a major hospital (if you're lucky), the post office, etc. This is discussed further in Chapter 10, "Planning an Office for a Startup Practice."

Should You Expand Your Present Facility?

It is rarely less costly to expand an existing facility. That, and other points (mostly problems) are listed below:

Feasibility

Will parking capacity meet legal requirements and accommodate the eventually larger number of patients and staff? Will obtaining your building permit depend on approval for your expansion from neighboring building owners and/or tenants?

Usually unfeasibility occurs because unplanned costs rise too high, as discussed later.

Unchanged Spaces for Practice Functions Will Become Too Small
Your aim to increase practice capacity by reworking existing space or adding new space could be blocked if you make too few changes to get the capacity you need. For example, if you add only exam rooms, then space in the waiting areas, preexam room, eyewear area, business office, eyewear delivery and adjustment area, and others could soon be inadequate—which means you'll need to expand again. This second project will greatly increase the total project cost, as detailed next.

Much Higher Costs
When further work must be done on a recently expanded office, costs for the total project will be much higher than expected because the new partitions must be moved to get the space needed for expansion of the unchanged areas that became too small. The second contracting and design cost would probably raise the eventual total to an unacceptable level. A new location might have been a much better choice.

The Direct and Indirect Costs of Down-Time
The loss to your momentum and reputation could be truly serious when you are closed, usually for weeks, during rebuilding. Your reputation could suffer if patients resent that you didn't arrange contingency care for them long in advance of the shutdown you knew was coming.

The direct cost of being closed is, of course, the lost income, some of which will be recovered if patients will wait. Patients with an urgent need (leaving town, a repair, contact lens red eye, pain, etc.) often won't wait, so income and probably some patients will be lost. Indirect cost will include potential new patients who go elsewhere because the other office is open.

The Cost and Misery of the Alternative: Remaining Open
Some doctors practice during the renovations, in the uninvaded spaces. The contracting is done in stages, which costs more as the contractor must bring back the same tradespeople for each stage.

Much worse is the construction work, (noise, dirt, disruption, etc.) adjacent to where you and others are working. This inflicts a truly miserable experience on your unsuspecting patients, you, and your increasingly unhappy staff. One doctor told me of the power saw howling on the other side of his exam room partition, while he shouted at the patient in order to be heard. When the saw stopped abruptly, he was still shouting. He vowed, "Never again!"

If you choose expansion to solve your problems and achieve your objectives, move temporarily to nearby vacant space and set up a bare-essentials practice. Then your phones are answered, appointments are made, emergencies and repairs are handled, and patients have someone helpful to talk to. A handsome sign on your existing, under-construction office would direct people to your temporary facility.

What Is Available to Rent or Purchase?
The availability of an acceptable location could limit or even kill the project. Location choices will of course be confined to available, acceptable alternatives. Those acceptable alternatives could include:

- Space on the retail level of a mall or smaller shopping center
- Office space in a low-cost building (usually to meet a tight budget)
- An existing home that you could rent or buy, and probably expand (rarely good)
- An empty or about-to-be-empty store

Describe your preferences to real estate agents specialized in professional space, and one or more bankers (who often are informed about available space). Be sure they grasp that you are a doctor, not a merchant, and the perceptions your facility must win from those who notice the exterior and those who enter. Try to find creative people who will recognize a novel opportunity if it turns up. Be sure they become aware of your need for:

- Visibility
- Appearance related to demographics of your patient base
- A particular size or space
- Parking, passing traffic, etc.

You will be educating the real estate agents (and they you), so they will be able to focus on the main points and the important subtleties of what you need.

Remember that unless you have a buyers' agency agreement (so you pay the agent), real estate agents are working for the seller or landlord and also for themselves (by trying to get a sale or lease at least cost to themselves, i.e.. as fast as possible). Through a buyers' agency agreement, which establishes that this person is working for you (and is paid by you alone), you can have a real estate agent's skill and knowledge on your side.

Find an agent who wins your confidence (ask around for references). Then hire her/him to help you find the best location. The fee could be worth every penny, and more than offset by your earnings from taking care of patients while the agent does the looking. An optometrist I know saved money by continuing to practice all day while an expert looked for his new location. He was delighted with the promising places she found, and was the obvious winner. But note that real estate agents may not know or choose to tell you of locations that are or are about to be available. That is why you should talk to several different real estate firms.

Don't misunderstand any of the above. Real estate agents are often good-hearted, reliable folk, but unless they're paid by you, their loyalty is likely to be elsewhere.

Use your free time (evenings, weekends, etc.) to look around. Drive and walk through areas you feel are promising, and note any signs offering sales or rentals. Ask at the local Planning Office about any buildings or developments that will be started soon. Find people likely to know about possible locations in the community, neighborhood, or area. Talk to other professionals as suggested earlier: other doctors, dentists, and lawyers, plus bankers, business owners, the Chamber of Commerce, and larger general contractors.

Unless you have good reason to be worried about the confidentiality of your potential plans, this personal exploration is usually worthwhile, and it could be very helpful if it leads to a top-notch location. Let people know that it's your success that forces you to find a bigger, better location.

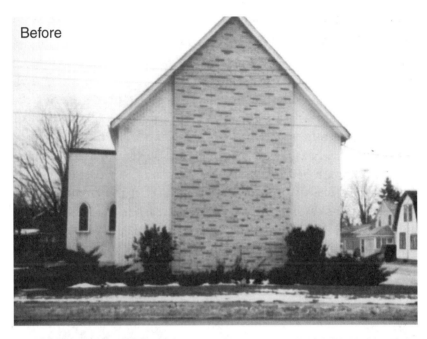

Before

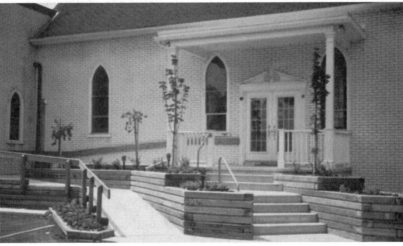

Figure 4–5   See page 39 for the AFTER picture of this rented church, remodeled for an optometric practice—a valid investment. The entrance on the side of the church was seen as so attractive that a wedding party used it for their formal photographs. (Reprinted with permission from Dr. Betty Fretz, Listowel, Ontario.)

Converting an Existing Building

This promising possibility requires some imagination—and some experienced advice. A former home, a bank, a restaurant, a church, and a recognized historic building have all to my knowledge been successfully converted for eye-care practices. See the photographs here, for some examples. You will probably know or easily learn of others.

There are hazards. A former home is often too small and is constructed with bearing walls that can add to the cost of conversion, made necessary by rooms that are often too small. Former service stations can be tempting as they are often on a corner, with acceptable parking. However, environmental law often requires that the land in which the gasoline storage tanks rested be replaced. A former bank usually has a vault that will be a bit costly to remove.

On the positive side, a former church can be ideal with its lofty ceiling, and usually has acceptable parking. Similarly, a free-standing former restaurant can have the space and parking that you want. Instruct your real estate agent to include buildings that served other specialized functions in the search for your new location.

Additional Advice

In all relocations, make a determined effort to do the following:

- Try to make sure that your present location won't be taken by another eye-care operation. Perhaps renew your lease and then sublet if your lease permits it. Check whether landlord permission to sublet is required in your lease, and if so whether it says, "Such permission may not be unreasonably withheld." At the very least, try to find the new tenant yourself.
- Do a great job of informing patients of your new location. Word-of-mouth within your practice is probably best, but will be restricted to those patients who visit you after you are certain of your new location. Give each of those a business card with your new address.
- Make sure that you send handsome announcement cards (in envelopes!). Don't send computer-generated letters to

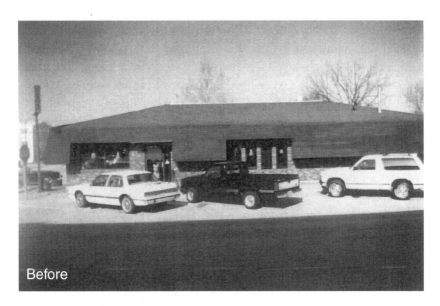

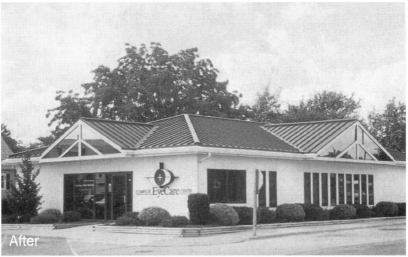

Figure 4–6   This well-located building (a former fast food restaurant) has good parking, but its former appearance rarely attracted attention, and when it did, it left weak impressions. Skilled planning and designing turned its weaknesses into strengths for a practice of optometry. (Reprinted with permission of the American Optometric Association. *AOA News,* August 1998; 8C.)

patients or strangers. They will be widely ignored, or even resented as more junk mail. Remember to enclose at least one business card with each announcement card. Announcing a move effectively is so important that you will be wise to be guided by practice marketing consultants.

- Make your new location easy to find—a fine, well-known building, sometimes called a "good address."
- If you erect or modify a free-standing building, be sure its exterior is visible to drivers and/or pedestrians, and that its highly noticeable, attractive appearance wins the right perceptions. Excellent signs are essential.
- Regardless of the distance you move, make your new location patient friendly (convenient and pleasant for patients). This well-known point involves:

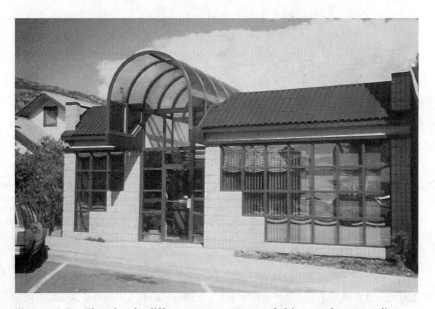

Figure 4–7   The clearly different appearance of this new free-standing street-front building designed for their practice of optometry makes it noticeable and capable of winning good impressions, such as with the canopy to the curbside, while distinguishing their practice from nearby retail stores and supporting their identity as doctors. (Reprinted with permission of the American Optometric Association. *AOA News,* August 1998; 8B.)

Your own parking lot, or at least generous adjacent or
   nearby parking
Ease of turning off and onto the access street
Absence of an inappropriate operation next door, or even
   close by
Handicapped parking at your entrance
Wheelchair ramps, and perhaps automatic or motorized
   doors
A weather canopy to your entrance from the parking lot
   and/or sidewalk

Take care of the many details of choosing, planning, and
marketing your location, as discussed in this chapter, and your
path to project success should be much smoother.

Own or Rent?

Will Rogers said, "Buy land—they aren't making it any more." Is
that good advice? As another wag said, "I can give you a definite
maybe."

Examine your advantages and disadvantages from owning
and renting the place in which you practice. Although your decision will occasionally be obvious, often it won't be.

When Renting is Better

Sometimes renting will clearly be the better choice— or it may just
appear to be. Renting will usually be your only choice when you
don't have all of the following:

- Enough money to buy real estate (land, plus a building)
- Enough money left to install yourself there to the needed
  standards
- Real estate purchase payment level close to what you would
  pay as rent (more on this later)

Remember that when you buy real estate, its purchase comes
before the substantial cost of installing your practice in your
empty building (a cost that also occurs with rented space). This

first expenditure (buying the land and building) is an investment in real estate that probably shouldn't be judged as an investment in your practice. From a financing point of view, analyze your real estate investment as a separate, perhaps nonessential venture even when the building is for your practice alone.

Your second investment will be for leasehold improvements that prepare the space for your use. When you rent, you won't face the cost of that first investment, the real estate, but you will need to pay for the second investment, regardless of whether you rent or purchase.

Between the two investments, your real estate and your practice, the "goose that lays your golden eggs" will normally be your practice.

If that first cost, the land and building (real estate) leaves you with too little money to install your practice well enough for its

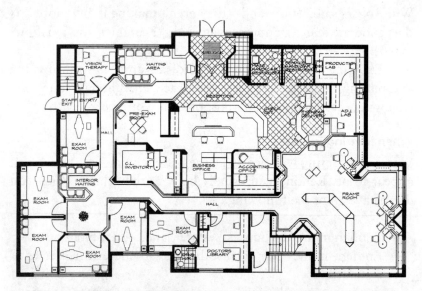

Figure 4–8   Designed to provide a much bigger facility and meet the objectives, needs, and wants of these doctors, this 4,283 sq. ft. building shows too many points of note to identify here. As you read Chapters 5 through 9, you will appreciate most of the doctors' choices. (Reprinted with permission from Drs. Steven Gander and Bruce Storhaug, East Grand Forks, Minnesota. Population 8,700 [over 80,000 in both cities].)

essential growth rate, you will need to rent, in order to concentrate your investment where it will pay off best for you.

Further, cost overruns, common in building construction (often for changes) can cause unexpected and potentially dangerous financing problems that are less likely to occur when you rent—although you should remember that cost overruns also occur in leasehold improvements.

Some successful private practice eye doctors find, particularly in their practice's middle life, that too soon after a good relocation, they are again hurt by a shortage of space. A relocation will usually be easier (though still difficult) when you are a tenant.

When you own your building and must again relocate, you have the added task of selling it (not to another eye doctor!), preferably before you purchase or lease another site. The sale of your building at a suitable price could be slow, as you look for a buyer who values space that was chosen and laid out to be best for an eye doctor's use and success.

If you conclude that inadequate capacity is likely to enforce another move too soon, you may want a larger space now (rented or purchased).

An Additional Move to Even Bigger Space Is Not Necessarily Bad

As mentioned earlier, some eye doctors, including those who own their buildings, view the need for another move as an acceptable and even welcome part of their successful, normal career path. They look forward to even more success in another new facility, confident that they will gain excellent benefits (well known to retailers and mall owners) from updated marketing and the public perception of a clearly superior operation that is implied by the new quarters.

As already described, a second relocation will usually be more difficult for an owner than a renter.

When Constructing a New Building is Better

Since a suitable, truly impressive, free-standing building is rarely available to rent or buy, and the benefits from having the right building are so important, your best, most powerful option could

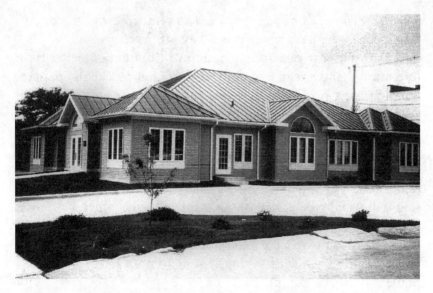

Figure 4–9 Despite being alone in a small community this doctor erected an impressive new free-standing building designed for his use located in the center of town, with its own and adjacent public parking. The result has more than justified his decision. (Reprinted with permission from Dr. Riley Uglum, New Hampton, Iowa.)

be to construct a building to meet your special needs. Even then, finding a good enough site can be difficult.

Your advantages from public and patient perceptions of a suitable building on a well-chosen lot were presented and discussed earlier. As the owner of the right building, on the right site, you can market the outstanding strengths of its appearance and convenience, as described next.

Appearance of the Building

Your building should present your eye-care practice as in the health-care field, professional, successful, notable, and (you hope) distinguished.

It is almost impossible to give you in words a good understanding of these outstanding eye-care practice buildings. A photograph can help, but not nearly as much as a visit where you can see and appreciate a colleague's new building and its right-

perceptions exterior. After a few such visits, you should more easily recognize an appropriate, impressive building, or visualize how a new one should look.

The following, including the next section, expands on and emphasizes points made earlier in this chapter. During visits or from photographs, note your perceptions of these buildings. Ask yourself if the buildings are highly noticeable, and present the previously listed, instantly recognizable evidence that is likely to generate an observer's perceptions of:

- A successful practice
- A doctor, not a merchant
- A doctor of firmly held high standards
- Excellent good taste

The exterior appearance of your building should also be distinctive. It should be instantly recognizable as different from (preferably better than) its neighbors, in a way that wins attention, and admiration for you as a successful doctor.

Appearance of the Site

Your site should win perceptions that convince the public and patients of welcoming convenience and high standards. These early positive perceptions can help to create the right mind-set in these people before they enter your building.

It will likely be easy for you to recognize an acceptable site (land, with or without a building on it). Its essential features will be:

- **Size.** Big enough for present and soundly forecasted future needs, such as building expansion and parking.
- **Visibility.** Open lines of sight to all passersby.
- **Accessibility.** Easy to find and to get to.
- **Good volume of passing car traffic.** But not moving too fast.
- **Easy for cars to turn in and out of parking lot.** Obvious.
- **Prestige location.** From association with other nearby buildings and/or health-care services. Or your building can create its own perception of prestige, particularly if it is not too close to other less impressive buildings.

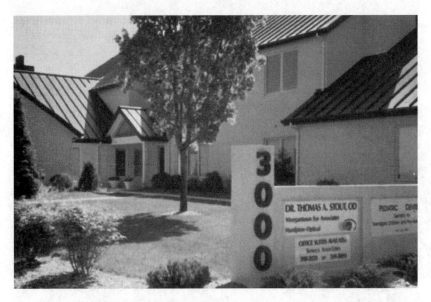

Figure 4–10 This practice made a highly successful move from down-town to the outskirts, onto the ground floor of a health-care building in the handsomely kept, prestige setting of a professional park. (Reprinted with permission from Dr. Thomas Stout, Morgantown, West Virginia.)

- **No wrong neighbors.** No operations that are dirty, noisy, smelly, messy, and/or attract people incompatible with your patient group.

The Right Reasons for Owning

When the real estate (building and location) will clearly be very good for your practice and represents a sound investment (because it yields its own acceptable return on investment), and when its purchase leaves you with adequate financing to install your practice properly, you will have very good reasons to own. Because values often go up, expecting a good eventual ROI from a real estate investment is not as risky as you might expect. But sometimes such a venture is not even considered because, without a thorough investigation, the prospective buyer expects that a sound ROI is unlikely, and thus dismisses the purchase as need-lessly risky.

Sometimes you can finance a real estate purchase with payments near the rate of monthly rent. In such a case, purchasing wins, as it gives you the big advantage of eventually owning a valuable asset.

You may want an asset/investment for your estate, particularly if you are unable, or it is difficult for you to buy life insurance. A doctor I know in that unwelcome position bought carefully selected real estate, including the building for his practice, and got protection for his family by willing it to them.

If after a thorough search you must conclude that no acceptable rental space is available, your only alternatives may be to own your space or to postpone or abandon the project.

If lack of suitable financing or something else forces you to rent, and you can't find acceptable rental space, look for someone with capital (such as an estate—ask your banker) who wants a good investment and sees your proposal as filling that need.

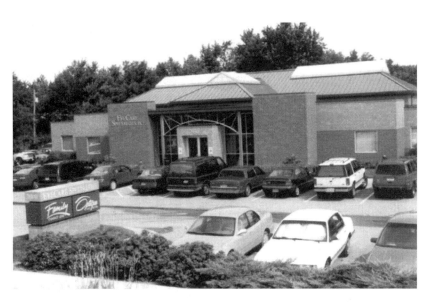

Figure 4–11 The impressive appearance of this large free-standing building, designed for their sole use, presents convincing evidence of success, high standards, and excellent taste, powerful contributors to the speed of practice growth. (Reprinted with permission from Drs. James Kirchner and James Devine, Lincoln, Nebraska.)

He/she erects the building based on a long-term (say, ten-year) lease from you, often with an option to purchase at the end of the lease, or if the owner wants to sell.

Don't neglect a thorough look at possible tax benefits from a real estate venture. Although tax gain may rarely justify a real estate investment, this information could help tip the balance in favor of owning, and guide your structuring of your venture's financial side so it attracts no more tax than necessary. Financial advisers should be helpful here.

The Urge to Own

At first glance, the urge to own seems such a sensible, secure, comfortable idea, that anyone opposed is probably against motherhood, and in favor of sin.

The urge to own may be instinctive. Some eye-doctor tenants in single occupancy buildings, or those considering renting in one, seem convinced that they should own it, even when that decision is financially questionable, or even contrary to logic (rational business analysis).

When they don't own, some doctors are reluctant to invest the substantial sum needed to install their practice well enough in their rented space. This reluctance can deny them the perceptions they need from patients and the public for an optimum rate of practice growth.

Their reluctance is understandable, since an unfamiliar major outlay can be worrying. But this view won't withstand scrutiny. Many thousands of retail business tenants wisely and comfortably make heavy investments in their leasehold improvements. They have confidence based on experience that, correctly done, the investment will pay big dividends. Further, leases in some major malls require retail tenants to do extensive renovations every few (three to five) years, because the tenant's greater success pays off for both the tenant and mall (the mall through percentage rent).

A doctor tenant may object to all this because of the urge to own. Some eye doctors seeking a better facility seem to view renting as "second best," a compromise acceptable only when owning isn't feasible. As noted earlier, a building is a tangible asset. If it will eventually be owned by the doctor, then perhaps renting a comparable building is not the best choice. However, such a comparison is valid only when the locations involved are equally good and there is financing available for both of the investments required.

Make sure that your urge to own is based on a proper analysis of your self-interest. As noted above, circumstances will dictate whether you will be correct to choose owning, or the alternative, renting.

Will My Real Estate Investment Pay Off?

Most serious investments, including real estate (usually with the exception of your home), are motivated by return on investment. In real estate ROI has three sources:

- Income produced
- Capital gain
- Tax benefit

Income Produced

Income produced is rental revenue minus costs. As landlord and tenant, you should find out the going rate for rent for your quality of space in your community. You should perhaps pay yourself rent at that rate. You will then have a correct revenue number for your accounting. A local real estate agent can guide you on the amount of this rent.

Your accountant should set up separate records for your real estate, so you will know your investment's return or lack of it. These records should be started soundly and early, and be properly maintained, regardless of whether you purchase an existing building or erect one.

If you wish to put up a building, a contractor should identify in a quotation the cost of the empty building as you would have received it from a landlord. This will permit you to examine the feasibility of your real estate investment before you commit to it.

After construction is completed, you should get from your contractor the actual cost of the empty building. Your accountant will of course need that cost to calculate the annual return or loss on your real estate investment.

Add up the cost of the land, the empty building, financing interest, legal and surveying fees, etc. Assuming that as the tenant, you pay triple-net rent that covers building maintenance and taxes (common in leases today), then the sum of the items above will be your total real estate cost as owner/landlord, correctly identified in your records as a separate investment. This real estate investment should have its own targeted, percentage rate of return, and a targeted time span for it to be paid off.

Tell your contractor that his reported empty-building cost must exclude all leasehold improvements needed by you as the tenant, for your practice. He/she may be familiar with this request. The leasehold improvement items for exclusion from building cost would include the practice's partitioning, plumbing, extra air conditioning and ventilation, specialized professional lighting and controls, etc. Your designer should be able to pick them out easily from your contractor's list of costs.

Now you can calculate the minimum rent you would have to pay yourself for the real estate investment to produce an acceptable ROI, or merely break even. You could then decide to set this minimum rent higher or lower than the going rate of rent for similar space in your community. The rent you choose will be a matter for study between you and your financial advisers, but the study should include the factual information below.

Annual rental revenue must cover the owner's annual financing and other payments for: the land, the building, financing interest, building management and maintenance (if paid by the owner), your return on investment, etc.

You and your financial advisers will decide how long you should take to repay your real estate investment (both borrowed and personal). The number of years for repayment will control the size of the payments in each year, which will influence the real estate ROI.

If the local going-rate rent doesn't at least cover costs and ROI, you are losing money. When this occurs, the owner usually sees it as problem. See "A Nonviable Real Estate Investment."

Capital Gain

Capital gain from building ownership is long term and cannot be known until the property is sold. However, it can be estimated at any time from known real estate market values. When the property is sold, the capital gain could range from excellent to disappointing.

Capital gain (and tax benefit) is rarely the prime reason for constructing or buying your practice building. There is an element of risk in capital gain forecasting, even when you have the advice of experienced real estate agents, financial consultants, bankers, accountants, and others.

The Tax Picture

This is a specialized matter that will depend on tax laws and regulations, and perhaps your personal or practice financial position. As noted earlier, your financial advisers should explore this with you.

A Nonviable Real Estate Investment

A real estate venture is normally declared "nonviable" when total net revenue fails to cover the costs plus a reasonable return on investment. One common reason for a real estate venture being nonviable is that the building is too small. Architects and real estate people say that too small a building will almost always be nonviable. Because eye-care practice buildings are often small (in professional/commercial real estate terms), you should investigate in advance whether your investment is likely to be viable.

I encountered one drastic case where an optometrist was so disappointed that his building was an unviable investment that he sold the building at a loss, sold his practice, and started a new practice in another community.

Nonviability is not necessarily an appropriate reason to reject owning your building. You could have at least two interesting alternatives:

If the income level from your practice, supported by this location, can be expected to substantially outweigh your projected losses on the building, your financial advisers might encourage you to proceed.

You could find a suitable tenant(s) and then put up a larger, viable building designed specifically for at least two suites. The tenant(s) could be chosen to be at least compatible with, and preferably helpful to, your practice.

If your proposed real estate project won't be viable, ask your management consultants whether you should:

- Give up the ownership project and find rental space
- Go ahead with the nonviable building
- Erect a bigger one

Is Freedom from a Landlord a Good Enough Reason to Own?

Some eye doctors say, "I must own my space so I am free from possible difficulties with a landlord." A landlord can indeed spell trouble for you. A difficult landlord might cause one or more of the following problems:

- Set unreasonable initial or renewal terms on space that is otherwise excellent
- Refuse to renew an expiring lease on acceptable terms
- Rent the space beside you to an undesirable tenant

However, the real benefits of freedom from landlord involvement must be weighed against your challenges and the potential downside of being an owner. Your choice between renting and owning should probably be based on the points discussed earlier.

CHAPTER 5

Design Criteria
for Most Clinical Functions

Your design criteria for the clinical and related support and management areas of your new office will come from your examination of each function to be accommodated. This process should offer abundant opportunities to strengthen your practice by upgrading patient services.

Your Mode of Practice

This book is directed mainly to those optometrists and ophthalmologists who have or want a private practice, probably with a broad range of services and functions. Other modes of eye-care practice will often need the same services as those presented here, but are not listed or discussed, even though many of the design ideas would be suitable for others, such as in an HMO or a clinic. You probably will have chosen your mode of practice before embarking on your choice of location and office design.

List Your Needs and Wants

Begin planning the accommodation of clinical functions in your new facility by listing your "needs and wants" in detail. In doing so, answer or consider these questions:

1. What present clinical functions (as they are now, or changed) will be needed?

2. What existing and predictable new functions, some based on new technologies, should be introduced—as for example may be needed in response to the U.S. government's document "Healthy People 2010"?
3. What space(s) will be needed for maximum capacity in the above functions?
4. What will the (new?) sequence be for all functions?

Accommodating Innovations in Practice Technique

Important new functions in eye-care practices, such as computer-assisted diagnostic procedures, are here already, and more are sure to come. New in-office surgical procedures seem quite predictable.

Vendors will usually be glad to reveal their planned introductions. In optometric practices, one important new service could be the presence of a surgical ophthalmologist, as discussed at the end of this chapter. Also, there are the growing administration requirements in dealing with insurance plans and managed care. You will be able to add to this list.

The expanding list of clinical and related management and patient service functions undergoing serious change at this time includes:

1. Preexam
2. Computer applications
3. Assistants' duties
4. Special testing and services

You and your designer must be sure that your list is reasonably complete, and that each function's procedures are properly understood.

To assess your prospective designer's ability to understand the functions and procedures you need, discuss with her/him the space and design needs revealed by your list of all existing, changed, and/or new clinical and related operational functions—your "clinical needs and wants." When you feel confident that you are talking to a suitably competent designer/consultant, begin the critically important analysis of the functional and space needs of each item on your list. This detailed analysis of all your clinical and related functions permits your designer to specify the clinical-side design criteria from which your plan will be developed. This analysis is thus an exacting task, crucial to project success.

Design Planning for Functions: Cost Related to Benefit

The validity of cost/benefit analysis for choosing among alternatives will be well known to you, as it occurs frequently when you discuss choices with patients.

The cost of each function-space must be justified by the benefits it delivers. This will control how much space to give to each listed function. For each such space you will need to know its:

- Contribution to patient care and welfare
- Contribution to the short- and long-term benefit of the practice
- Cost of inclusion in your new facility

Space costs money, whether you rent or own. For some eye doctors, the cost of space, and the need to make the best use of money available, could limit or block the accommodation of some worthy functions that would benefit patients or help in managing the practice. Your advisers should be familiar with the realities and predictable changes in your profession's practice, as a base for their recommendations regarding space per function.

Here is another key point about cost. Your planning decisions that are based on cost (including space and design decisions) should be respected by your designer and/or adviser, even if you disagree. These consultants should present their point of view, but leave the decision and responsibility for the decision with you. It's your money, and your level of comfort with risk.

Make those decisions carefully. Your negative response to cost, while understandable and reasonable, could be seriously damaging to the achieving of your objectives. This point is so important it deserves this emphasis here.

Most of the clinical, management, and other nondispensing functions and areas are listed, discussed, and analyzed in this chapter. The clinical service design criteria that follow are in the sequence usually encountered by full-service patients.

Area Visible Inside the Main Entrance

Most eye doctors now want some kind of open design to welcome patients and visitors, an attractive vista of activity and service destinations, usually including:

- Reception station
- Waiting room
- Eyewear delivery, adjustment, and repair area
- Contact lens supplies station (in a contact lens pod?)
- Eyewear area (preferably not located so it is dominant)
- Patient restroom (and possibly other destinations)

Grouping service destinations for visibility and a sense of convenient availability will sometimes be limited by the size and shape of the space, but in any circumstances, skill will almost always be needed to do it effectively and attractively while taking the minimum space needed.

Open design helps win the perception of being user friendly. The level and quality of light, the sense of space, the accessibility of service destinations—all tend to build patient comfort, confidence, and interest.

In an open design arriving patients are directed by staff, floor finishes, lighting, and minimum signage. The rare patient intrusion into the clinical area is usually controlled easily by staff.

Some doctors still favor a door between the reception/waiting area and the rest of the office. It is a time-honored design that yields firm control over patient access to the "inside." With a closed door in place, the doctor can move freely through all inner areas without risking eye contact with patients waiting or at reception, who would often expect to be greeted by name, and perhaps expect some time-consuming chat.

Also, reception staff sometimes complain that with open design they occasionally have difficulty with a lack of phone privacy. This is discussed in a following section, "Reception Station: Outer Business Office."

There are usually ways of getting reasonable levels of patient control and staff privacy in open design, with minimal risk of damage to the patient's sense of being welcome. Be careful and creative about this, to protect the valuable patient pleasure of feeling wanted and important. For staff privacy, have an adjoining "inner office" (also discussed later). For the comfort and control of waiting patients, present absorbing videos, mostly about eye care, that hold their attention.

An open front suggests a less formal, more relaxed, with-it atmosphere, implying an enjoyable experience to follow. This desirable perception can please almost all patients.

Access Approaches to the Inner Functions

Access routes (hallways) to inner functions should be interesting, never boring. Changes in direction and width, with points of interest, stimulate patients and create positive perceptions.

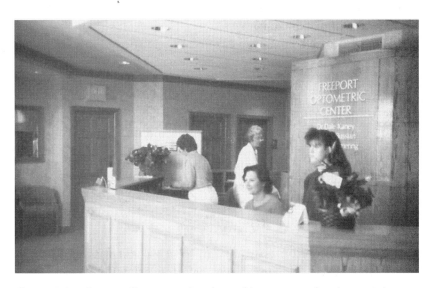

Figure 5-1   **If you assign several tasks and have space for them at the main reception and checkout stations of a quite large practice, there should always be one or more staff there to promptly receive patients and attend to their needs. (Reprinted with permission from Drs. Dale Kaney and Todd Bussian, Freeport, Illinois.)**

These access routes (sometimes a corridor) should have cool medium lighting that changes in level and color to announce arrival at each new area. This is widely used in malls and walk-through exhibits. By stimulating alertness as each new area is approached, this lighting can trigger and heighten interest in a way not usually noticed by the patient. These techniques can convert a corridor walk from a nothing experience to pleasure.

Reception Station: Outer Business Office

This station is where a patient first meets staff. It should be as friendly and welcoming as its personnel. It should be truly near the entrance, and enable staff to see most of the following:

- The entrance and patient coat rack
- The waiting room (all of it, if feasible—perhaps by the use of cleverly placed mirrors)
- The eyewear delivery, adjustment, and repair area
- The contact lens supplies display, and the C.L. Information Center (if you have it)
- The entrance to the eyewear area (usually not critical)
- The patient restroom

"Reception," where people are warmly welcomed and get a caring response to their needs, should usually be a nerve center and often a checkout station. Its staff should be able to:

- Keep patients feeling comfortable and welcome
- Give immediate assistance when needed
- Work efficiently
- Adapt to changing responsibilities

When a reception assistant can see a patient waiting for help at a visible service position (eyewear delivery, contact lens supplies), that patient can be greeted and given timely assistance. That is why it is so important that at least one assistant be available at reception at all times. This is valid in almost any practice, but particularly in a larger, busier one. This rapid-response service delights patients by honoring their importance. It will be available most often when a number of tasks are grouped at reception so that it becomes an outer business office, often used by several assistants at the same time, and thus frequently well staffed.

When telephone privacy (mentioned earlier) is needed, avoid having a barrier across most of the reception counter. Transfer sensitive incoming calls to the adjacent, much more private inner business office, where sensitive outgoing calls are made. The perception of "welcoming" that comes from openness at reception is far too valuable to be given up for telephone privacy that can be obtained in other, only slightly less convenient ways.

Design reception to reduce the risk of others overhearing sensitive conversations with patients. Consider installing one or more privacy cubicles near reception for this and other purposes. In some practices, these cubicles would be used prior to service, to discuss with patients the details of insurance plans, Medicare, etc. And they could be useful for checkout (often done in this vicinity) so a patient can be seated, particularly to write a check.

Except in large practices, have two stations, "checkin" and "checkout," at your outer business counter, separated to yield some privacy, and located so patients tend to arrive at the correct one naturally. In large practices, checkout is sometimes in a nearby, separate location.

A computer printer could be at reception, between the two stations. One set of the (essential?) signal lights that silently tells staff when and where they are needed should of course be in this area.

Patient Record Files

Computerized filing of patient records is growing irresistibly. If you don't have it, surely you should plan and design for its almost certain installation as part of your project.

Some computer consultants predicted paperless offices. In fact, computers generate more paper than ever before. So you will probably need to file many paper reports, memos, etc.

Your computer files of patient records will have paper or tape backup, sometimes a legal requirement You will probably want tapes stored at home (for security against fire, etc.) daily, weekly, monthly, or annually. Fast access to backup records may be a consideration.

Do regulations specify kind of storage? In the exam room, will computerized patient files appear on a screen or as a print-out? How will you input new patient data? Are you as a doctor required by law to have tamper-proof records? If so, are computer files acceptable, or must they be on paper?

If you now have computerized filing, or plan to introduce it when you move, do these files contain complete clinical and treatment (e.g., dispensing, contact lenses) records, or just the financial history? This will affect office organization and, to a lesser degree, design.

Decide where your traditional paper files should be. They will usually need to be immediately accessible at the outer and inner business offices, or perhaps in an adjacent, separate file room. This is discussed later in this chapter, under the heading "The Role of Computers: The Scope of Change."

Other Matters Affecting Front-End Design

The eyewear area is sometimes located close to waiting, usually to encourage patients to enter. Even if located here (see discussion of this location in Chapter 7), it should be staffed at all times so it will not be a responsibility of reception staff.

In one interesting idea, an assistant is assigned to each patient on arrival, to serve that patient in all assistant tasks throughout the practice, now and on subsequent visits. In this program, assistants might wait for their patient at appointment time, at the front end.

Telephone Placement to Avoid Voice Mail

Most doctors have been told by patients and know from personal experience how annoying it is when their phone call is answered by voice mail. I've heard that an increasing number of doctors are reorganizing their reception of telephone calls to avoid having the caller reach voice mail.

In your new office, try to have enough telephones at usually manned stations within easy earshot of each other at the front end, so all incoming calls can almost always be answered by a person, not a machine.

Have at least one more of those telephones than you have incoming telephone lines. If you have one or more separate, unlisted lines for making outgoing calls, have the number of front-end phones at least equal the number of incoming lines.

Your management consultant could help you with this.

Inner Business Office

This important room is sometimes omitted, and frequently is too small. Doctors have often told me they regret that their inner business office isn't big enough to handle all its functions.

The size of the inner business office will usually depend on three factors:

- The size of the practice
- The space needed for the functions to be performed there
- The cost

Again, its size should allow for substantial growth. It should be big enough that it won't feel crowded when it has work stations for at least half of the staff and temporary help, and seating for others who could be there for coffee and/or to communicate (an important need in any size of practice).

There should be one assigned work station and chair for each assistant who regularly uses the area for routine tasks, and one for sporadic major jobs (which may take several hours or days). Smaller or less frequent tasks could be done in unassigned positions. Most if not all of these work stations should be arranged so the work can easily and routinely be interrupted and resumed, as will happen often.

The inner business office could be used and/or may be needed for the following functions:

1. Computer input and printing beyond those listed below
2. Accounting, including:
   - Accounts payable
   - Accounts receivable (and collections when needed)

- Production of financial reports
3. Nonaccounting recordkeeping procedures
4. Doctor-requested assignments
5. The use of business machines—fax, copier, etc.
6. Letter production and dispatch (newsletter?)
7. Sensitive phone calls
8. Recalls (phoned or mailed)
9. Follow-up phone calls
10. Business filing (sometimes also patient record filing)
11. Informal or impromptu staff–doctor meetings

If there is a practice manager with a private office (as in a big practice), some of these functions would be accommodated in her/his office.

A coffee maker for staff could be in the inner business office, so staff would remain available in a central, accessible place while having "a cuppa." If the coffee maker is also for patients, put it near the door to the reception area, or perhaps put another one in the waiting room. (A practice in an upscale area serves tea in fine china to patients in the waiting room.)

As feasible, the inner business office and the reception/outer business office should be located next to each other and designed with lines of sight so the reception counter is easily seen from some key stations in the inner office. A door or opening is needed between them for immediate access. The visibility of the reception counter will permit staff in the inner business office to respond promptly to an unattended patient at reception. Since patient needs are always top priority, the assistant in the inner office would leave his/her task to look after the patient, or at least alert another assistant to do so.

The inner office needs enough sound privacy so that normal conversations cannot be overheard by patients outside. This includes the privacy needed for those sensitive phone calls. Conversations in the inner business office can also gain privacy by being masked by music from speakers directly above the counter at the reception desk.

Doorways in the inner office should, as feasible, lead to the following areas:

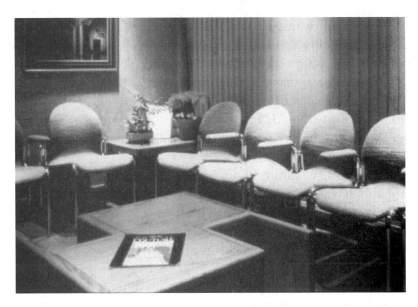

Figure 5–2 Main waiting room in an upstairs practice in a small town of mostly modest-income people. Its restrained attractiveness is evidence of the doctors' standards, which supports the practice against competition and pays their patients the compliment that they merit this level of practice. (Reprinted with permission from Drs. Joseph Kronick and Morris Hazan, Hawkesbury, Ontario.)

- Reception/ outer business office as noted above (top priority)
- The file room (if there is one)
- The diagnostic areas close to assistant tasks (preexam, etc.)
- Perhaps the eyewear area (not if, as is usual, it has its own full-time staff)
- The manager's office (if there is one)

Main Waiting Room

Decide on the seating capacity your practice will need after 5 to 10 years of speeded-up growth. Have extra seating for patients who arrive as a family or with an attendant. Except in a startup, you will already know approximately how often this happens in your practice.

Less main waiting room seating will be needed if you have (as you probably should) adequate internal waiting areas (discussed in the section that follows, "Internal Waiting").

You may feel that you need a truly big waiting room, because your present one is often crowded (a sign of inadequate patient-service capacity, and/or inadequate internal waiting). Remember that with your new increased practice capacity, fewer people should be forced to wait.

If your new waiting room is crowded much of the time, you probably have one or more persistent bottlenecks in patient flow (usually they are obvious), which must be reduced or, where feasible, eliminated. Adequate, balanced capacity at all patient services should minimize bottlenecks, improve patient flow, and hold down waiting times.

Bottlenecks that can't be eliminated will tend to be at exam rooms because of inescapable additional time required by an occasional patient, or an emergency or some other unavoidable situation that delays the doctor. As detailed in the next section, these quite common bottlenecks caused by doctor delays should usually be handled by placing patients in internal waiting, not back in the main waiting room.

In your waiting room seating, chairs are best, followed by benches and then sofas. Studies show that unrelated people will almost always fill vacant chairs first, then the ends of a bench or sofa. Chairs (not deep) with arms are better so people who can't move easily can more readily get themselves in and out. When benches seem unavoidable because space is seriously limited, they are a little more acceptable if they have individual positions separated by arm rests.

In a specialized practice such as pediatric optometry, or sometimes because it is the "style" of the optometrist, a homey-look waiting room may be wanted—perhaps with big chairs, a sofa, and even a fireplace. This living-room type of waiting room usually requires much more space than is needed for the more traditional room. This can be a problem if it either takes too much of the total office area or reduces the waiting room's capacity. However, doctors who have such waiting rooms report that patients like them. If it's your style and you feel you can afford the space, go ahead.

Regardless of the details of how you plan your main waiting room, patient perceptions of it should be, "This is a friendly practice run by caring, capable people."

Your new waiting room should provide:

- *A children's play station.* This can be a small enclosure, well stocked with toys, and with carpeted floor and walls, often in a corner, enclosed by a barrier one foot high and wide. It works best with quite young children, who are often the hardest to control. Or, the play station could be a child-size desk or counter with at least two seats (or something more creative). A play station is a must. It gives these children (potential future patients) a pleasure they remember, while also pleasing parents and siblings. Adults often appreciate your kindness to children, and the absence of disturbing child activity that is often brought on by boredom.
- *An information center.* Main and internal waiting areas are ideal information centers. Many patients want to know more about their eyes, vision, and health care. That interest extends over a wide range of eye-care services and material. Also, patients are usually happier, and waiting time passes faster when they are watching something interesting.

  Audio-visual presentations are best at providing combined information and entertainment. All waiting rooms (main and internal) should have a suitable place for an appropriate size of TV monitor and an individual or a central VCR for appropriate video stories. Potential presentation uses of video and/or computers are described in Chapters 7, 8, and 9.
- *A patient restroom that is wheelchair accessible.* Installed as a courtesy, this should be visible from the front, but not exposed to all in the waiting room. It may strike you as an avoidable expense. But remember the occasional times when you needed a restroom and had trouble finding one, or were embarrassed to ask in a busy, crowded place. It is particularly

helpful with seniors and children, but greatly appreciated by patients of all ages.

The law in your area may not yet require "wheelchair restrooms," but more and more jurisdictions do require it. You would be wise to make all your rest rooms wheelchair accessible in any new or renovated installation.

The Impact of Computerized Refractors on Preexam Procedures and Your Profession

The design criteria for preexam areas, covered in the next section, may need to be rethought in response to computerized refractors that obtain subjective findings by patient interaction with a computer that drives a refractor. They are said to take less than fifteen minutes per patient and will probably get faster. The operation of such an instrument and its time needs will affect the design of the preexam/data-collection facility (and perhaps of the exam room). Information for guidance on this will be available from the manufacturer, colleagues, your professional association, etc. By the time you read this, much more will be known about computer-controlled refractors and their impact on patient care and on the operation of an eye-care practice.

Preexam Design Criteria

There are persuasive reasons why preexam data collection is increasingly done by suitably trained assistants, such as a COT (Certified Ophthalmic Technician) or a COA (Certified Ophthalmic Assistant). As one prominent educator explained, third parties who pay in part for eye-care education, and also for many eye exams, are increasingly reluctant to pay eye doctors to be collectors of data when:

1. Teaching an assistant to do preexam data collection takes far less time than is needed to educate an eye doctor.
2. Instruments with an increasing range of functions are now judged to be reliable and accurate, making it easier and even more acceptable for appropriately trained eye-care technicians to do preexam data collection.

The usual locations for preexam data collection in eye-care practices seem to be:

1. In a separate, dedicated preexam room.
2. In the one of a doctor's two exam rooms that he or she is not using at the moment, pre-exam date collection in a different room each time is made feasible by advances in portable, handheld instruments. This can be a welcome space saver in the practice.
3. In the exam room by the doctor as part of the exam.

Your designer will need answers to these four questions:

1. Will more than one dedicated preexam room be needed?
2. Will some or all preexam be done in an exam room that the doctor is not using at the moment?
3. If preexam will be split between the dedicated, and temporarily empty locations, which procedures will be done in each place?
4. Because some new technologies (e.g., the "Epic" system) may take more time with some patients, will an interior waiting area be needed there?

Preexam timing is important to patient flow. It will change considerably as faster and better instruments continue to be introduced, and better techniques and organizations are developed. The facility should be designed to accommodate expected changes, particularly in technique and organization, so the preexam timing matches or is faster than doctors' scheduled clinical appointments.

New instrumentation will rarely require changes in the design of preexam and exam rooms, such as different shapes or sizes, as manufacturers will avoid this for marketing reasons.

More than one preexam room may be needed when:

- Preexam consistently takes longer than the usual scheduled patient time in the exam room. This can occur when only one preexam patient can be served at a time—for example, when privacy is required while a case history is being taken. (Perhaps do this in a private, front-end cubicle?)

- In a multiple doctor practice where each doctor has a pod (a grouping of diagnosis-related functions including preexam—more about pods later), so that each pod has its own preexam operation.

In a busy practice, on-time flow of patients to the doctor could deteriorate when only one preexam patient can be served at a time. A second preexam room might be needed, or some portable preexam procedures might be moved to the doctor-free exam room.

To get good patient flow, the preexam assistants usually organize their operation so their timing coordinates with the doctor's and takes less time than the doctor will spend with the patient. This should make bottlenecks rare in preexam, as should new multipurpose instruments that offer improved efficiency and thus speed.

Obviously, you will try to find instrumentation with capacities that match your forecasted needs. If you know that your preexam capacity will eventually become inadequate, you will want to plan for this need.

You may feel that you should have a second preexam room, in spite of the cost of another set of instruments and tables. That cost can be acceptable, if not attractive, compared to the intolerable condition of doctors waiting for patients.

To plan for the design of your preexam space, decide first:

- Will privacy be needed?
- What procedures will be done in each preexam room or area?
- Who and how many assistants (or doctors) will do each of these procedures?
- How many qualified preexam assistants must be on duty at a time?
- How much time will be needed per patient (for an average case and for a more involved one)?

Get planning guidance from your own experimentation, contact with colleagues, and survey data from your professional association, instrument manufacturers, or elsewhere as available (see Chapter 14).

Some doctors use a wide range of procedures in their preexam data collection. They have the necessary numbers of assistants and instrumentation and are usually working with a considerable volume of patients. In such a practice the scope of preexam usually results in substantially less doctor time per patient. This style of practice is favored by some doctors as a means of serving their large number of patients and others who prefer a big solo practice. The latter group seem convinced that their methods should become the standard, and that their kind of practice will maximize their personal income.

In such a practice the preexam space will of course be much larger than usual, with an appropriate office layout (three, four, or more exam rooms will probably be needed, and a facility that yields efficiency for a relatively large staff).

Preexam seems to be an eye-care function in transition. Before choosing the functional and efficiency criteria that will control your preexam design specifications, ask at least a few colleagues about their experiences, and their predictions for the future of preexam in your profession. Then, decide how your preexam space(s) should fit into your reorganized, expanded practice.

With your designer, decide how much preexam space you will need for:

- Results that meet your standards
- Timing for flow that will help you avoid a bottleneck here
- Capacity that allows for the forecasted growth in patient numbers
- A worthwhile contribution toward your objectives

The design criteria for your preexam facilities should emerge from: your answers to the above questions, data you obtain from third parties, and the knowledge of a suitably experienced designer.

Interior Waiting

An internal waiting area is a kind of reservoir ("staging position") that takes care of the almost inevitable fluctuations in patient flow that occur in most established practices. Internal waiting is also usually needed for the eye dilation period, even with doctors who want to encourage dilating patients to visit the eyewear area.

A busy practice with capable staff, balanced capacities per function, and well-organized patient flow will still encounter some unavoidable patient delays between functions. As noted earlier, some bottlenecks occur at the exam room when a patient's care takes longer than allotted, or when an emergency or other urgent matter takes unscheduled doctor time.

Internal waiting near the exam or other procedure rooms is often also needed for friends, relatives, or professional caregivers who might accompany a patient, but cannot go with them for some clinical functions because there isn't enough space in the procedure room, or it isn't appropriate for them to be present, or the doctor prefers to work one-on-one with the patient.

Patients tend to be happier in an internal waiting area than they would be back in main waiting. Even though they are again waiting, they see themselves as doing better than the less fortunate patients who are still "out there."

The obvious locations for internal waiting areas are:

1. At the exam room(s), for patients after preexam and during dilation, and for those who are with them.
2. Just outside the eyewear area. This is needed if the eyewear area is full, or if there is too little space inside for extra people who are with the patient.
3. At the contact lens area, particularly if yours is a busy contact lens practice.
4. Beside the "delivery services" (eyewear delivery, adjustments, and repairs—often called "dispensing") for patients waiting to be served and extra people with them. This internal waiting should often be the largest, since even when delivery is by appointment, patients who need an adjustment or repair usually arrive on a random basis.

As noted earlier, each internal waiting area should have audio-visual, often left running in a busy practice. This is a superior way of informing patients about eye care and vision, emphasizing proper eye care, and explaining practice functions still to come. More and more videotapes are becoming available. Where appropriate, videos in different languages will make you look special.

As you know, time spent waiting can become more acceptable, or even welcomed, when patients perceive that professional information on vision and eyes is being well presented as an appropriate part of their care. If some major news or other event is on, the monitor should be capable of being switched to TV.

If one patient needs to be shown a particular video, this is best done in a private place such as a consulting room. But, in the absence of a properly equipped private room, internal waiting might be the only place available. The videos you have prescribed for this kind of private viewing should be easy to call up on a computer, either the same computer as the one that shows the tape, or a computer than controls the tapes shown on the VCR.

"Internal waiting," also called "internal seating," is usually accepted as imperative in all but startup and early-days practices. It should not be deleted for reasons of cost.

Assistant/Technician (A/T) Work Stations and Their Locations

You already know that your assistants/technicians are vital to your success. Their role is growing in most practices. Their expanding formal education, continuing education courses, and on-the-job training all point convincingly to further growth in their status and areas of responsibility.

If possible, each A/T should have a "base work station." Each station will usually need at least a desk with the items for the job(s) to be done there. Each A/T should list the things they want. You and your designer should then review each list with the A/T who wrote it.

Each A/T's base work station should be close to where most of their work is done. Sounds simple. But many A/Ts perform multiple tasks, with varying time demands, in numerous locations. The location of their base work station will sometimes have to be a compromise. That is why the A/T, you, and the designer should choose its location.

As feasible, keep A/T stations near each other. Your aim is to have one or more small clusters of A/T base work stations plus the few that must be relatively isolated. The benefits of this are discussed below.

Groupings of staff stations should make it easier for one of the staff to break away from a task to do the more important job of attending to a patient. These clusters also yield improved communication among the staff there and will make it more likely that the area will be manned when one of the A/Ts is doing another task elsewhere or is in the rest room. As previously noted, this pertains particularly to the reception/outer business office and the adjacent inner business office.

Since each A/T's base work station location will depend on the site of his/her most time-consuming tasks, organizing who needs to be where for what should be a team responsibility. The team should of course include you, the A/T involved, and probably your most experienced A/Ts.

To decide on location and design criteria for each A/T's base work station, your team should:

1. Develop a comprehensive list of their present functions.
2. Tackle together the harder job of predicting their expanded, modified, or new tasks.

In making the second list, anticipate the addition of one, and perhaps two more doctors and extra staff, plus the further reorganization of your operation at a later date in response to growth.

Encourage innovative planning in the new accommodation needed for your staff.

Each solo A/T station should almost always be in one of the three following places:

1. Inside the procedure room to which the A/T is mainly assigned
2. In a small office or cubicle next to, or near that procedure room
3. In a knuckle (a wide spot in the access route) near the procedure location

In talking with your assistants of all sorts (not just technicians), find out if any would prefer to stand at their work station. It may surprise you that in one busy practice most assistant A/Ts (not technicians) chose to stand. They felt that standing all day was less tiring than getting up and sitting down so many times.

Many variations are possible in assistant tasks, work stations, accommodational needs, locations, staff preferences, etc. As a result, your staff organization may differ greatly from others. For that reason I prefer not to recommend a formula. Develop your own together.

Two interesting ideas for assistant services in your practice are presented next.

Interior, Manned Patient Support Stations (One or More)

Located beside a major interior waiting position (particularly the one at the exam rooms), this support station would have one or more assistants (possibly technicians) who have regular operational duties, but whose dominant responsibilities include:

- Making patients feel comfortable and cared for, not alone and isolated
- Moving patients
- Explaining what is happening
- Introducing the patient to the next A/T who will serve them

Just by being available, sympathetic, and helpful, this assistant can:

- Please and reassure patients
- Answer questions they were reluctant to ask, or thought of after seeing the doctor
- Respond to patient personal needs such as the restroom or an urgent telephone call
- Just be someone for a lonely or apprehensive patient to talk to

This interior, manned patient support station should have an assistant present most of the time. Otherwise it becomes much less effective, and a potential waste of space.

It can be in a knuckle, but will usually be best in a good-sized cubicle beside the busiest internal waiting area. There could be a writing surface, a computer terminal, filing, a phone, signal lights, etc. To encourage easy communication a fence (low partition) would separate this area from the adjacent interior waiting.

Practice benefits will be:

- Patient admiration for this easy to use, caring, helpful service
- Smoother patient flow resulting from escorted patients
- All the operational tasks that assistant performs there or close by
- Reminding staff of caring for patients, the underlying function of the practice

Assigned Assistants

As mentioned earlier, one innovative optometrist assigns an A/T to each arriving patient. This A/T remains with her/his patient throughout the visit, and as possible, on all subsequent visits, doing all the assistant-technician functions. This way the patient and A/T tend to develop a warm relationship, which builds patient confidence and pleasure. It also overcomes the negative patient perception of being "just another pair of eyes"—a feeling that can come too easily in a big, busy practice.

These A/Ts would need extensive training for acceptable competence in all patient care duties. Most will be happy to get this training. More A/Ts might also be needed. These A/Ts might have their base work station in a front-end cubicle or small office where they would be most readily available to greet the arriving patient and to work with the patient in relative privacy when needed.

Doctors' Pods in Multiple Doctor Practices

The term *pod*, as used here, identifies a group of related functions that clearly belong together. In a multidoctor practice each doctor would have his/her own pod. Each doctor's pod could be almost identical (no "master bedroom" concept) and would usually include:

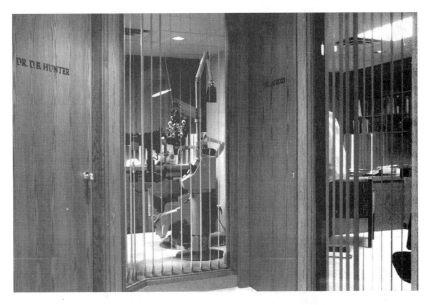

Figure 5–3 Typifying one part of a doctor's "pod," the adjacent examining rooms provide efficiency for the doctor moving between them. The small window walls permit doctor awareness of and then response to the activity level, and let patients see in and thus have a perception of openness. (Reprinted with permission from Drs. Donald Hunter, James Ross, Douglas Turnbull, and Ronald Gaucher, Regina, Saskatchewan.)

- Two or more exam rooms
- An interior waiting/information area
- An assistant's station, cubicle, or room

and perhaps:

- The preexam operation for that pod only
- One or more procedure or treatment rooms as needed
- The doctor's private office

All routine diagnostic procedures will almost always be available in each pod. Procedures that are only needed intermittently would be located between the pods, as convenient to all of them as the total office space configuration allows.

Here's how it works. The patient is escorted to her doctor's pod. Inside the pod the waiting area and all routine clinical services

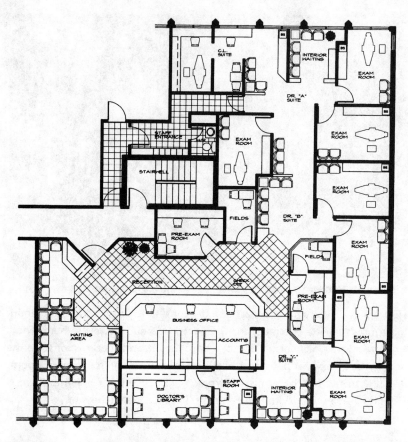

Figure 5–4 **Combining three practices, these ophthalmologists accepted an early version of the "pod-per-doctor" design concept with each doctor having two exam lanes and an adjacent internal waiting area. They have since considerably enlarged their contact lens pod, the original of which is at the top left of the plan. (Reprinted with permission from Drs. Dickson, Allin, and Kidy, Brampton, Ontario.)**

will be just a few steps apart. The doctor, usually with a full-time A/T, will have a sense of being in better contact with the patient and will work comfortably at an optimum pace (with very few delays) while enjoying the efficiency.

That efficiency, normally inherent to the pod layout, can yield greatly improved patient care and flow, to the delight of doctors and staff in multidoctor practices. In such practices without the pods, the sustained higher demand in a less efficient layout can yield a less productive operation.

Each pod will tend to give patients the pleasing and familiar impression of "*my* doctor, in her/his practice, taking care of *me*." This strengthens the bond between patient and doctor and for the patient, gives the potentially intimidating big practice the friendlier feeling of a smaller office. You will recognize that the pod layout comes from the clinical layout and efficiencies of a single doctor's well-designed office.

A downside could be a reduction in communication among doctors and staff outside the pod, who would encounter each other less often.

Multiple Exam Rooms per Doctor in all Sizes of Practice

Today, eye doctors usually insist on having two or three or more exam rooms (lanes). Here is an incomplete but still convincing list of the reasons why you will need at least two rooms from the start of your practice.

- Efficiency in the use of doctor time, as each new patient is always in place and "prepped" as the doctor enters the room
- Privacy for the taking of an appropriate patient case history by a qualified A/T
- Location for preexam procedures that can now be done by a qualified A/T, using portable (handheld?) instruments
- Location for contact lens recheck by an A/T, unless there is a separate contact lens exam room, ideally as part of a contact lens pod (see Chapter 6)
- Location for emergency care as the need arises

Examination Rooms

Doctors usually tackle this with justified confidence and convictions. Today, most doctor/owners want two or more exam rooms per doctor.

Almost all are satisfied with their findings in a mirrored room, rather than one that is sixteen to twenty feet long or longer. Mirrored exam rooms save money on space, and release it elsewhere for other present or future practice functions. Good designs have space-saving techniques such as this that don't threaten success or comfort.

Exam rooms must not be too small. Beyond the important questions of examination result validity, and the need to accommodate present and future equipment, there is the potential problem of doctor stress from many hours in a room that feels small. This causes some doctors to "escape" as often as they can, unaware of their frequent absences or even their reason. The stress of too many hours in too small a room can affect mood and/or alertness, which can prejudice patient care, and perhaps harm doctor health.

As noted, your exam rooms should be designed for present and future equipment. Changes to the sizes and shapes of existing exam rooms to accommodate new diagnostic units such as computers are unlikely, as the renovation costs would make the items too expensive for many possible buyers.

The physical dimensions of the exam room, and the design factors that create the feeling of space, need skilled attention. Good specifications would be a room nine or ten feet wide, and about twelve feet long, with a side entry door to save steps for the patient and the doctor, and with lighting, décor, and other elements that make it feel larger.

A window wall with blinds, or made of darkened glass, between the exam room and the access route (corridor) lets the doctor see out at any time, and outsiders see in when blinds are open or lights are up. It will also help to make an exam room feel bigger to the doctor. Also, with a window wall doctors and staff are less isolated—more aware of office activity. One doctor said, "When I see things getting very busy, I cut down on unnecessary conversation and make sure I lose no time." A window wall anywhere in the practice yields a more open, less hidden feeling for patients who then perceive you as an open person.

If your busy practice is a local center to which people with emergency eye problems are likely to come or be sent, consider having one exam room for emergencies and other intermittent situations needing fast attention. With emergency patients, this room will be used for care and/or triage (deciding which patients you can treat, what you must do, and which must be referred to a hospital immediately—that you would then arrange).

When you are needed in your emergency exam room you can explain the situation to your present patient, who then simply remains in the exam room you are using. This eliminates the awkwardness of asking your present patient to leave so you can bring in an emergency patient. A patient may dislike being uprooted for any reason, but may be satisfied (and impressed) to have you leave the exam room briefly to take care of an emergency—a recognized worthy purpose.

An appropriately equipped "emergency" exam room would be set up for special procedures such as removal of a foreign body. It could also be used for "red eyes" or any other patient need for prompt attention.

Consider having a "wheelchair exam room." In one project, local media emphasized this aspect in their TV and newspaper

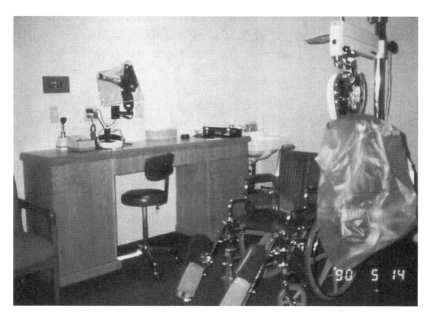

Figure 5–5   Wheelchair examining rooms are a service for handicapped patients, and a strong public relations move. When this location opened, a local TV station chose this item to feature in its story. (Reprinted with permission from Drs. Mark Mather and Brian Davis, Muscatine, Iowa.)

stories for its human-interest appeal. There is a type of examination chair that moves away to accept a wheelchair. Until the wheelchair room is used frequently for non-wheelchair patients, you could park your wheelchair there with the door open, so passing patients know of this service. Remember that better accommodation for the handicapped is required by law in a growing number of jurisdictions. If this is not yet law in your area, shouldn't you act before the law requires it?

Ambulatory Surgical Center (ASC) Room

If you will need an ASC room, check whether your designer has the experience to design it or will need guidance.

Minor Surgery Room

If you are an ophthalmologist, or an optometrist with an ophthalmologist associate, you will need a minor surgery room. The criteria for this service must be carefully analyzed by you (the doctor) and your designer. It will help if the designer has experience in this area, regarding the key elements of space, lighting, fixtures, etc.

Special Testing Room

By definition, this room is for patients who need special diagnostic testing—fundus photography, corneal topography, pathology screening, fluorescein angiography, and more. Its use can be expected to keep changing. It should obviously be big enough for all its present and predictable procedures, despite space and cost pressures to keep it small. Make sure that it is well ventilated and doesn't seem confining. A window wall to the corridor would help, but wouldn't be appropriate for field analysis which is also in the selected-patients category, but is usually given a room of its own because it requires light control, and perhaps extra sound isolation.

In larger offices, put the special testing room centrally among the doctors' pods.

Vision Therapy (Developmental Vision Care) and Sports Vision

Many optometrists and ophthalmologists seem to view vision therapy with mixed feelings, although it is widely acknowledged as meeting a recognized need. A few practices get deeply into vision therapy, others offer active but limited service, and some omit it because of its unfortunate reputation among some doctors—that it is difficult and yields a low return. For some doctors, it is outside their comfort zone. Each eye doctor will decide on his/her practice's involvement in vision therapy.

Sports vision is newer but has been around for quite a few years, and also seems to be restricted to practices where the doctor has the knowledge, interest, and aptitude needed to be comfortable with the service.

If you will be providing one or both of these services, tell your designer early. A designer experienced with eye doctors' offices will usually know about the space needs for vision therapy and/or sports vision operations. But techniques used in these practices can be seriously individualized.

Give your designer a detailed description of the techniques (procedures) you want in your vision therapy and/or sports vision operation. Or, if feasible, direct your designer to a facility that approximates your ideal.

Here is a suggestion for doctors who want their vision therapy and/or sports vision practice to be recognized and accepted as a community referral center for this service. Install the practice in a small, former factory building (6,000 to 10,000 sq. ft.) that has been empty for some time, on a lot with plenty of space for outdoor activity and parking. Its location and long vacancy might yield low rent, or a modest purchase price. Enough office space should be available for eye exams and other clinic functions plus a working room for each of your associates (psychologist, teacher, etc., and key assistant/technicians). You will need its typical factory high ceilings for some processes, for example gross motor training. Of course, before proceeding, you will need to find out the cost of adapting the building for your use.

The suitability of this facility would tend to impress all professionals in child education, plus parents and even their children (the patients). In sports vision it would be similarly impressive.

Location is always important, but a marginal location such as this could work—the patient numbers for your success will depend on referrals, not passersby (although passing traffic could still help). Try for a well-known street, so patients will find you easily.

Obviously, before beginning this venture you would need dependable assurances from those listed below of approximately how many patients per month they would refer to you. Their answers, and sincerity if you can judge it, would control whether you proceed. They are:

- The local optometrists and ophthalmologists
- Principals, teachers, and psychologists in the local schools
- Local related organizations and individuals such as parents, social workers, school coaches, police (juveniles dept.), Lions and Rotary clubs
- Family physicians
- Any others you can think of

Some eye doctors (particularly optometrists) seem reluctant to refer a patient to another eye doctor in their profession, but this should recede as their confidence in the service rises, and patients are returned after treatment.

Consulting Room

Few practices have a consulting room. Cost/benefit studies usually give it low priority. However, the ancient slogan for Packard cars that urged, "Ask the man who owns one" could also apply to an eye doctor's consulting room. Those who have one report that this pleasant room, usually with a window, an informal grouping of comfortable chairs (no desk), a coffee table, plants, and appropriate lighting, has a friendly, relaxed atmosphere well liked by all who use it. A memorable consulting room shows the doctor's commitment to doing all things well.

The consulting room would be used for:

- Special case presentations to the patient and/or family
- On a later visit, discussion of patient and/or family concerns or interests that at this time won't require any exam room procedures
- Surgery consultation
- Meetings with important visitors
- Possibly occasional kinds of eye-care service, such as low vision
- Seeing detail persons, supplier reps, etc.

Without the barrier of a desk, the consulting room is friendlier than the doctor's private office, which might be untidy if the doctor has an unfinished project. The other alternative is of course the more formal exam room, which lacks the relaxed feeling of the consulting room and may not be large enough for a family.

Some doctors have such a full schedule that the idea of being able to spend time in a consulting room would amuse them. But even they and key staff could use a consulting room, possibly routinely, and certainly when an appropriate need arises, provided that this happens often enough to justify it.

Doctor's Private Office

Despite how little you may use your private office, it should usually be a priority item. If nothing else, it's a private place to make or receive sensitive phone calls. Even the busiest doctor benefits from having a place that is hers/his alone.

In the absence of a consulting room, the private office is the appropriate place for interviews with colleagues, staff, job applicants, your accountant, other health care professionals, etc.—not only for the sake of privacy, but also because needed information is available there. It can be used for projects (professional, personal, or community-based, such as a charity drive) that will need to be interrupted, leaving the room a little messy.

A private office is a place to relax between patients—which is not available elsewhere (other than the restroom!). One doctor asked that his office be soundproofed so he could "go there and holler" to relieve tension. Where appropriate, a private office should have a window. Doctors also like an adjacent, personal restroom, often with a shower.

In a multiple-doctor practice, harmony may be promoted if each doctor's office is the same size, but perhaps decorated to individual taste. Or, it may be accepted that the senior doctor will have a "master" private office.

Where space or budget are tight in multiple-doctor practices, a larger room may be used by all of them, with a desk for each doctor. This saves cost and space, while giving the doctors a place for their professional library and doctors' meetings, but it also reduces individual privacy.

The only factors that could eliminate the justification for a private office are that there is not enough space, or that the cost would be too great.

Practice Manager's Office

A well-qualified practice manager can be central to large-practice success. Despite this, some doctor/owner(s) of large practices prefer to handle management themselves. These doctors tend to feel that this keeps them in touch with the management side of their practice. (Of course, the doctor could be kept "in touch" by a practice manager who has proper communication skills.)

Doctors who favor having a top manager seem convinced that doing management tasks during the day reduces their time for patient care—which only they and the other doctors are qualified to handle, and which produces the income. And they want their evening tasks confined to those that only they can do and that hold the most promise for the practice.

A practice manager's office should be where her/his presence will yield the most for the practice. The best location will thus be at the front, within sight of the busiest stations, patient arrival/reception, eyewear delivery-adjustment and repair, checkout, and contact lenses.

A doctor may want to reserve such central space for services that produce immediate revenue, but having a manager there will usually assure even greater earnings. A window wall (with motor-driven blinds for privacy) between the manager's office and the front end will reduce the manager's isolation. It also lets the manager see the strengths and weaknesses of the operation, and respond to patient problems, staff shortages, bottlenecks, etc. This location will also be convenient for staff and patients who need or wish to talk to the manager.

The manager's office should be large and attractive enough to convince patients who see it that this is a place where important things are done well and pleasantly. Try for two doors, one to patient reception, and the other to the inner business office.

Staff Room

A staff room will be justified by its functions. It is not a luxury. Its presence and size will depend on its use, the numbers of doctors and staff, and the total office space. It should permit the expanded staff to meet comfortably for numerous valuable purposes, including those increasingly important education/training sessions. Assistants and technicians need these sessions to help them handle the increasing clinical responsibilities that you and they will probably want. As feasible, training should be held in-office for convenience and efficiency, and so demonstrations can be done using existing equipment and office layout.

Where space for a staff room is a problem, you may wonder if you could make your inner business office large enough for staff meetings. This is almost certain to be unworkable because space is almost always at a premium in the front end.

Because a staff/meeting room will be used intermittently, and not for patient services, it can, if necessary, be remote from the main staff work stations (perhaps on another floor). However, if it is isolated from the action, its use for coffee breaks could be a problem, as staff there wouldn't know about serious unattended patient needs. Although staff in such a room could be alerted to problems by phone, it's usually better when an assistant on coffee break sees the need directly and responds at once. Staff absences for coffee breaks can be avoided if you and your staff agree on location and priorities.

Staff coffee is usually needed in several places: the staff room (for use during meetings), the inner business office, and the production lab. The inner business office location is usually best for assistants and technicians because, as noted above, it then becomes feasible for a "cuppa" to be interrupted to respond to an unserved patient need. Your decision may affect your design criteria.

Storage and a Storage Room

A principle governing storage effectiveness is, "Store things at the place of first use." Keeping supplies at or near the work stations where they are used has obvious benefits. But cupboards, shelves, and drawers cost money—the usual reason why this valuable storage principle is often ignored in new facilities.

Before you drop the idea, though, think of the cost over the life of the practice of all the time your staff will spend going to and from their work stations to retrieve supplies.

Many years ago my wife and I reorganized our kitchen so everything was within arm's length of where it would be needed. The results were a delight of speed and ease. (In our kitchen, we had an advantage you won't have in your new space. There was no cost, because adequate shelving already existed.)

The design of storage units is also important. Shelf depth must be adequate for the items to go there, but not be excessive. Vertical distance between shelves can be adjustable, but not the depth (front to back). Similarly, with cubbyholes, width but not height is variable.

Tell your designer the dimensions and quantities of items for storage at each work station. Your more experienced staff can usually make excellent lists of these supplies. They should also choose which items should be at the convenient, accessible heights, not too far above eye level and reasonably above floor level.

One technique for localized storage is building a partition to be a "storage wall." These units replace cabinets that can be more costly for the same storage capacity. Normal partition width is about five inches. Increasing this to about fourteen to eighteen inches would yield floor-to-ceiling storage, with counters as needed. The storage and the counters could be accessible from either side of the partition. Storage walls need considerable space (as do cabinets), and they have the potential drawback that they are relatively immovable. But they probably offer the most generous and convenient storage.

Cupboard shelves on rollers are very good. They pull all the way out like a file drawer, so items at the back won't remain unseen until moving day. They're more expensive than the usual fixed shelving, but they offer storage for a wide variety of items. And when the shelves are on rollers, your staff will find that working with the high and low ones is easier because they can be pulled all the way out.

Despite the foregoing, a storage room is usually justified. Doctors have told me that even when the practice has good amounts of work station storage, they occasionally need a storage room to be used for:

- Supplies inventoried in large quantities, including stationery forms, brochures, etc., that are much cheaper when an annual supply is purchased.
- Bulky items, such as spectacle cases
- A place where incoming shipments can remain unopened for check-in at the most convenient time

When you have adequate storage at work stations, a remote storage room could be acceptable, even on another floor, since it will be visited only rarely. However, your storage room should usually have an appropriate, planned size and location, not be some leftover space labeled "storage room" regardless of its location or size.

The Role of Computers: The Scope of Change

Several long chapters or a separate book could be written about patient record filing in doctors' offices today and in the predictable future. As noted earlier, discussion of it here is largely confined to its impact on the planning and design of a new facility.

Choose your new facility's patient record filing system early in planning, since installing any system can involve a sizable investment and considerable time. Changes in record filing can be expected to affect your office design.

New filing options abound. If your patient records aren't computerized, you probably should be updating your knowledge of this well before planning your new office. The sooner you consider computerizing patient records or updating your present system, the more time you will have to research your options. Well before giving serious thought to a move, consult colleagues and appropriate computer service vendors about all aspects of filing patient records.

Paper filing, although still used to varying degrees, is becoming no more than backup to the computer records, and even backup is now often computerized (put on disk daily for remote storage, etc.).

Any book, chapter, or section of a chapter on filing should be written by or with a computer application expert, experienced in "Information Resource Management" (IRM) of health care patient records. I am not thus qualified, but I want you to have a list of some decisions about patient record filing that you may face, some of which could affect office design:

1. If you use paper filing, which system? Stored where?
2. If you use computer filing, will there be paper backup? Stored where?
3. About input:
    *   Will it be done by the doctor in the exam room, or by whom?
    *   Will all input be typed? Where?
    *   If input is verbal, will it be direct to the computer, or taped, or will it be written and transcribed later—in which case where will this be done?
4. Will access to a patient file be on paper or a computer screen:
    *   When needed by the doctor or assistant in the exam room?
    *   When needed by an assistant at a telephone, or any other time it is needed (the lab, the inner office, etc.)?
5. Where and by whom will the following computer procedures be done:

- Adding to records for existing patients?
- Practice management records and reports?
- Recalls and follow-ups?
- Research about the practice, or a patient?
- Financial accounting and tax records?
- Financial collections, etc.?

6. What are the legal requirements about protecting backup records against loss due to fire, flood, etc.? Off-site storage?
7. What safeguards against improper changes of records are required by law?
8. Where are the printers located?
9. If files are on paper, how much more than present space will be needed?
10. If you plan to continue paper filing, temporarily or long term, will you maintain your present system or install a new one? How will you accommodate the much larger numbers of records?

Switching to another system of paper filing will introduce potential difficulties. Before computerization, paper filing system competition led to many innovations, but now you may encounter problems getting supplies for some of those earlier sophisticated paper systems.

To start a design, your designer must know how you will handle all your patient record procedures, including filing. Your designer should respond to these needs, making sure the most important bases are covered in the most cost effective way for the system you have chosen.

Efficiency from Flow

As covered earlier, efficiency from good patient flow comes mainly from having the right patient capacity at each routine clinical function. No further discussion of that point should be needed here. Below are some of the other basic factors of good patient flow.

Locate practice functions to reduce doctor and staff walking time. Doctors and staff should walk the least because their time is a direct cost to the practice, and the doctor's applications of time affect patient service capacity. Pods, and/or two or more exam rooms per doctor, are good examples of reducing time lost to walking for all concerned.

As a matter of courtesy and convenience, also minimize patient walking. This is valuable in all practices, but it probably is only critical in a geriatric practice.

In the usual practice serving an average mix of patients, there should be appropriate design elements and service aids to help those patients who have problems walking.

As noted earlier, a doctor's pod yields diagnostic area efficiency through contributing to flow by being self-contained. The patient is only involved in the practice traffic when approaching or leaving the pod.

Patient movement and flow through the practice are best with a large core area, inside an encircling pathway. This needs a wide, rectangular space. Narrow rectangles or "L"-shaped facilities can be good, but permit less efficiency from flow.

With a pathway around the core, almost all patients move in the same direction. This gives them a good feeling about their progress through an interesting practice, and a perception of reduced crowding. In other words, the circling pathway pleases patients while improving flow.

As already noted, efficiency for patients and/or staff occurs when front-end functions, reception and inner business office, waiting, eyewear delivery, and its adjustment lab are grouped. Staff see when they are needed and can respond easily (with the fewest steps), as well as quickly.

In any shape or size of space there will be a limit to the number of function areas that can be adjoining. Spaces that are reasonably close and sequential will sometimes be the best result available.

Individual preferences of doctor and staff can be a factor in designing for efficiency and flow. Does the doctor like being visible outside the clinical area? Is he/she more of a hands-on or hands-off person throughout the practice?

Sometimes there is a design need that introduces a flow and efficiency problem. A practice with two widely separated patient entrances (street and parking lot) that must both be visible and controlled from reception can produce less effective flow or less efficiency. Also, a design dictated by space configuration may require some patients to move against the flow.

Efficiency and flow are truly important, worthy design targets. But they will rarely make or break the financial feasibility of the project. Where you can choose an adequate sized rectangular space, as close as feasible to a square (such as when you erect a new building on a big enough lot), you should get the best efficiency and flow. But you can still do quite well in a space with a less ideal shape.

For Optometrists: Accommodating an Associated Ophthalmologist

Until recently few optometry practices included the services of a surgical ophthalmologist. Although this is still not common, there is a growing trend for optometry services and those of a surgeon ophthalmologist to be available in a shared facility owned by the optometrist.

Because the functional and financial arrangements vary a lot, you will probably want to get guidance from a suitably experienced third party (colleague or consultant).

The big, often motivating advantages for the surgical ophthalmologist are:

- A good relationship with the optometrist
- An existing, properly staffed eye-care practice, in a facility of suitable quality
- A known good volume of eye-care patients
- Minimum investment to get started in the area.

The last is one of the stronger reasons why more ophthalmologists than before are interested. Even when an established ophthalmology practice is nearby, a doctor from that practice or an outsider might want to take advantage of your opportunity.

If this idea is attractive or just interesting to you, then during the earliest days of planning a practice move, you should start exploring it (before someone else does). If there is any interest, you and the ophthalmologist should have plenty of time to develop ideas for your future collaboration, long before you need to finalize the planning of your project.

Perhaps you should have an informal meeting with an ophthalmologist to whom you now refer patients, to at least introduce the subject. Explain that you are in the early stages of planning a much larger, better facility, maybe even erecting a new building. Does he/she have any interest in sharing your space (renting space from you) for a specific time per week or month? A suitable management consultant would improve on that idea. His/her guidance could put you at your best in your opening conversations with this ophthalmologist. Also, as always, talk to colleagues who have done this.

The accommodation needed for an ophthalmologist in your practice will range from the use of existing spaces to the provision of a pod that is almost always designed for the needs of both of you. The pod cost would usually be prohibitive if it is to be used by the ophthalmologist only, for only one or two days per week or less.

Once you and the ophthalmologist(s)have agreed on the idea of collaborating, and on the rent, you will want to discuss choice of space, its location, and its design. Your designer should then be brought in to work with both of you on the points that are pertinent in the circumstances—design criteria, cost, timing, design ideas, and more.

CHAPTER 6

Design Criteria
for Contact Lens Services

Contact Lens Pod

Your contact lens patients should be cared for in an impressive operation clearly specific to and appropriate for this major component of ophthalmic care.

Try to group your contact lens functions in a pod (a suite within a suite), for efficiency and patient perception of its importance. Then choose:

1. What established functions (updated, or as is) to include
2. What innovations to introduce
3. The location of the pod in the total suite

To serve your expected volume of contact lens activity, the pod may contain the following function areas and/or items, some of which would be combined depending on patient numbers. These areas are listed, and then discussed below.

1. A room for exams, rechecks, or problem solving where the doctor and/or senior contact lens assistant/technician ("A/T") would do appropriate procedures
2. A contact lens information center (room), for interested non-contact-lens patients
3. A contact lens introduction area where new contact lens patients get basic information about contact lenses

4. A contact lens patient instruction area
5. A contact lens patient training area
6. A delivery station for new and replacement lenses
7. Supplies station and display
8. A combined staff area (office), and where needed, contact lens lab
9. Doctor's diagnostic contact lens inventory (if all contact lens patients are examined in pod exam rooms)
10. Contact lens inventory for delivery to patients

Each of these function/areas or items is discussed below. But first, consider the following further points about contact lens pods for possible inclusion in your list of design criteria.

Staff specialized in contact lenses should always be available for fast response to patient arrival and needs. A pod will have assigned staff, with base work stations there.

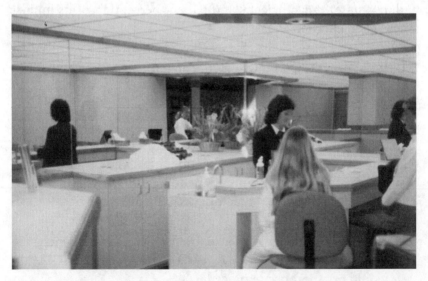

Figure 6–1   This contact lens pod area has multiple stations across counters and enough staff so that instruction, training, and delivery can be done at the same time. Patients are on high stools, with staff standing. (Reprinted with permission from Drs. Mark Mather and Brian Davis, Muscatine, Iowa.)

If feasible, the pod's display of supplies and the information center should be visible to patients as they enter the practice, and to assistants at reception.

Usually, all arriving patients, including those for contact lens service of any kind, should report in at the practice's main reception station. This will help to avoid confusion and to establish patient control. Patients needing C.L. services would then be escorted or directed to the pod. With the pod located near reception, this frequent patient transfer would be relatively convenient and efficient for patients and staff.

If you want separate reception stations (a practice with a large C.L. component), install a carefully operated system of staff communication and recordkeeping to avoid these problems.

Backup glasses for contact lens patients, an important part of the service, should be selected by the patient in the practice's eyewear area, to which they would be escorted by a C.L. assistant. Follow-up service on backup glasses would be done at the practice's "delivery, adjustment, and repair" stations. The patient would be directed there from main reception or the CL pod, and if necessary would return to the pod after the spectacle service.

Contact Lens Exam Room

An exam room in the pod is a convenient, impressive, efficient, and often delay-free way of delivering clinical care to your contact lens patients. It is particularly valuable in a practice that serves a significant number of these patients.

The contact lens exam room would be manned as needed by a doctor or senior contact lens A/T, or one followed by the other. Each would, of course, do the work for which they are qualified. This would include:

- A complete exam if this is consistent with office routine, and when you know in advance that this is a contact lens patient
- Contact lens fittings and follow-ups
- Contact lens patient problems and/or concerns, or immediate action situations

It has been my experience that in practices with a moderate to substantial volume of contact lens activity, this exam room justifies its existence while showing these patients your commitment to serving them.

Contact Lens Information Center

This is a newer concept, for practices that get many phone and in-office inquiries about contacts from strangers or the practice's spectacle patients. These people can be invited to have a free or low-cost session in your information center.

On arrival at the pod, these potential contact lens patients would have a brief discussion with a contact lens A/T, and then be seated in the information center, an attractive small room inside the pod. There they would see appropriate videos. The patient should be provided with a pen and paper for notes and questions. The offer of a cup of coffee might create a more relaxed atmosphere.

If feasible, the information center should be visible to the reception station, to increase the low level but necessary supervision. The information center could have glass or window walls to give a sense of space and openness. They will also be needed to permit the pod staff to respond as necessary to a recognized need. Your staff would of course recognize when an assistant should also be in the room.

Following the video presentation, the contact lens assistant would return to answer questions and, within reason, win a friend for the practice.

Contact Lens Introduction Area

When you examine new and perhaps repeat contact lens patients, you will almost always want to give them introductory or updated information about contacts and fees. Presenting a sufficiently complete story can be time consuming, but you will want it done effectively, and it will save staff time in the long run as described below.

You would cover the key points briefly, but in a busy practice the full introductory information would probably be presented by an assistant in a separate space, and to save that assistant's time you may prefer to have this important information presented, at least in part, by video. The videos should cover all the information that C.L. patients need about contacts, except the "instruction" (care) and "training" (handling), which are discussed in sections that follow. The video would be clinical, based on patient welfare, not a promotion of a product or service. (Promotion has its place, but not as clinical information.) Video suits this job because its story doesn't vary in completeness and emphasis, as discussed in the next section.

You will probably want a small, separate video room, which could be the just-discussed contact lens information center. A video room would keep the C.L. introduction presentation from being cut short, and also keep it from tying up you, your exam room, or your "instruction" room (presented in the next section). In this introduction video room, after the contact lens assistant's opening remarks, the patient would see videos, again with pen and paper for notes and questions.

Contact Lens Patient Instruction Area

Instruction of patients is indoctrination aimed at compliance, presenting the patient's responsibilities, and the correct ways of dealing with all aspects of C.L. use except the physical handling of the lens (placement on the eye, removal, cleaning, etc.—this is "training" and is covered in the next section).

In many practices, instruction and training are combined during a single session in one location, which is fine until that location can no longer handle the number of patients. With separate rooms for these functions, both can be in use at the same time.

Because instruction, indoctrination, and compliance are so very important to contact lens patients and thus to the practice, the strengths of video presentation could be critical to both. Video instruction also yields the efficiency of less assistant/technician time, but its biggest benefits by far will be on the professional and legal side.

During instruction, even the best A/T could on occasion be distracted by such things as an unanswered phone, an unmet

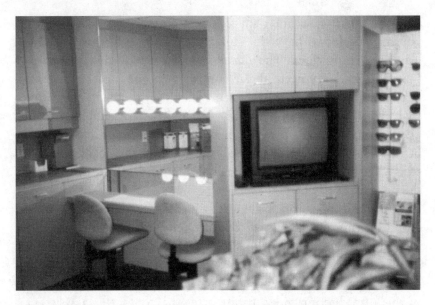

Figure 6–2 Contact lens instruction on the right and training on the left are separated by a stub wall. Training is done with assistant and patient on the same side of a counter facing a mirror. (Reprinted with permission from Dr. Gene Zackowski, Creston, British Columbia.)

urgent problem, or a demand for service elsewhere. Then, understandably, some part of the story might be omitted or underemphasized.

A tape always tells the same complete story, with the same points of emphasis. In the unlikely event that a patient sues you for inadequate instruction, your tapes will prove that nothing was omitted. Further, you and your staff will have the professional satisfaction of knowing that your patients receive complete and identical instruction, every time. During this instruction video, the patient would again have pen and paper for notes and questions, to be dealt with by a contact lens A/T immediately after the video session.

Tape vendors are slowly increasing their range of products, but you still may not be satisfied. You may want to make your own tapes, which you might see as an interesting, attractive challenge. At least you may want to add your own introduction and conclusion to the purchased tapes.

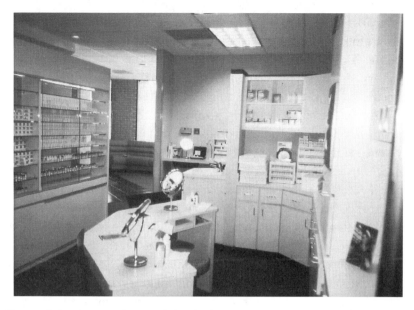

Figure 6–3 Contact lens training is done across a counter with patient and staff seated. (Reprinted with permission from Dr. Arnold Stokol, Richardson, Texas.)

Contact Lens Patient Training Area

"Training" covers all pertinent contact lens handling procedures, from the less extensive with disposables, to the more demanding with longer-wear custom lenses. It is done by an assistant.

Your designer will need to know:

1. Is patient privacy preferred (one patient being trained at a time)?
2. Do you or your assistant/technician want to face the patient across a counter or be on the same side, facing a mirror?
3. How many stations will you need for simultaneous training, in whichever setup you prefer, either one-on-one privacy sessions, or sessions with multiple patients?
4. Do you plan to use this location to deliver new contacts to patients, or will you want a separate station(s) or position(s) for this?

Most doctors have well-established procedures for contact lens training and delivery, but will welcome this opportunity to update. Tell your designer the details of the C.L. training and delivery systems you want in your new office, and how many patients you want to be able to serve at a time.

A contact lens training room should win perceptions of devotion to hygiene and a strong sense of fashion. A perception of hygiene reinforces patient indoctrination about the care necessary in all handling of their contacts. A perceived fashion atmosphere appeals to most contact lens patients, as their sensitivity about appearance probably led to their decision to have contacts.

Lighting at training should yield a relatively shadow-free face and should be either unobtrusive or attractively noticeable. Patients who prefer to use a horizontal mirror for inserting or removing their lenses like additional light through that mirror which is usually built into the counter. "Color temperature" lighting here will give patients a healthy-looking complexion.

If feasible, there should be three built-in counter mirrors at each station, one vertical, one horizontal, and one angled, to meet all patient preferences. The mirror angle and working position should feel right to the patient and have doctor approval. Small adjustable-angle mirrors are less impressive and sometimes hard to use.

Delivery Station for New and Replacement Lenses

Should you afford space for a station dedicated to delivering new and replacement contacts, or should this be done elsewhere in the pod, perhaps at the training counter? Also, some doctors feel that their patients prefer to have these lenses sent to them at home. However, other doctors want the patient to make this visit as it will be an opportunity for:

- Checking the patient and stressing their need for their contact lens eye-care program
- Reinforcing compliance with prescribed lens-care procedures
- Being sure the patient has backup glasses

This delivery station could be a small counter for seated or stand-up use at contact lens checkout, visible from the entrance and reception. This works particularly well when you have a C.L. pod, since a C.L. assistant/technician will then almost always be present.

You may be tempted to use that counter for contact lens pod reception and payment of fees. But, as noted earlier in regard to reception, doing so might reduce patient control at main reception, and might also be confusing to some patients and to staff responsible for fees.

Supplies Station and Display

This is where patients get contact lens supplies. Because it brings your contact lens patients into your office often, this service increases their chance of receiving valuable ongoing professional care and supervision from your C.L. staff. Some doctors see this as so important that they price these supplies near cost, in order to be below local competition.

Your full range of contact lens supplies should be presented attractively and conveniently in a handsome, properly lit showcase at contact lens checkout, both of which need to be visible from and near to reception. Considerable inventory of each product should be on the display, with backup supplies nearby.

The patient would pick up the items needed and take them to a contact lens assistant/technician for checkout. If the display is locked (which it should not be unless this is clearly necessary), the patient would be served by the contact lens A/T. Patients arriving at reception for C.L. supplies (probably their first such visit), would be escorted or directed to the C.L. pod, and an assistant there informed.

Combined Staff Office and Contact Lens Lab

Contact lens lab functions are needed less frequently now and usually require little more than a few feet of well-lit counter where, for example, an inspection and/or adjustment of the lens can be done.

That lab is not a good place for the contact lens inventory that is used in prescribing, since it should be as close as practicable to the doctors' exam rooms (see the discussion of this in the section that follows). The replacement lens inventory could be in the contact lens staff office or work area.

A staff office for contact lens A/Ts makes a lot of sense. It should be central in the pod and have low partitions for awareness of and prompt response to patient arrival and needs, while permitting good communication between visible staff. The C.L. staff office should have at least one phone, staff work stations, files, a computer terminal, signal lights, operating supplies, and more.

Doctors' Diagnostic Contact Lens Inventory

In a practice with multiple exam rooms, where contact lens patients might be examined in any of them, doctor-use C.L. inventory should be as close as feasible to the exam room doors. This is efficient for doctors or assistants obtaining lenses for a patient. Placing that inventory in all exam rooms would be more convenient but costly, and because a patient's interest in contact lenses isn't known in advance, inventory in only one exam room would be a gamble. C.L. inventory for doctor use in only one exam room would only work where there is one doctor with a single exam room, as in a small or startup practice.

This contact lens storage unit should also contribute appropriately to your marketing-by-perceptions, through its visibility to patients in the nearby internal exam-room waiting position. You have probably seen that people waiting notice and probably get perceptions from any activity in their vicinity.

Patients in internal waiting can be impressed by your contact lens inventory in its professional-looking, eye-catching display. These displays can reinforce patient impressions of your strength in this branch of your practice, and your dedication to patient service with contacts. Also, the noticed activity of a doctor or A/T in leaving the exam room to get these lenses will reinforce patient perceptions that this is a doctor's office.

Again, this display should be well designed, well made, and well lit (to your standard of excellence). Labeling will tell people what is there. One or more back-lighted photographs would add clarity, interest, and impact. This display, which must attractively house a quantity of blister packs and vials, will be a challenge for your designer.

Contact Lens Inventory for Delivery to Patients

Obviously this should be close to the place where it is needed, which will usually be the delivery station for new and replacement lenses. If it is also close by, the staff office is a good place because inventory management would be easier with the staff often there.

Staff Response to a Contact Lens Pod: An Anecdote

One manager of an excellent pod so much enjoyed her scope of responsibility and the pleasure she and her staff had in smoothly serving an outstanding number of patients per day, that her loyalty to her operation led her to reject a big salary offer elsewhere. She loved how well things worked in *her* pod and had seen the lesser CL setup that the other doctor felt was just fine.

CHAPTER 7

Eyewear Area Design Criteria

What "Dispensing" Means Here

Although readers familiar with this book's subjects would expect frequent use of the word "dispensing"—for example in this chapter—it will occur rarely because of its common use to identify any of the numerous eyewear functions. Here it will usually mean "all of the dispensing functions." For clarity, this book uses more specific terms that relate to each of the functions as they are presented in their separate chapters. These functions are:

1. Eyewear presentation (the main subject of this chapter)
2. Eyewear area management (included in this chapter)
3. Lens application presentation (see Chapter 8)
4. Eyewear delivery, adjustment and repair services (see Chapter 9)
5. Prescription lens production (Chapter 9)
6. Production lab management (Chapter 9)
7. Any other aspects of a full service eye doctor's dispensing operation (Chapters 7, 8, and 9).

Eyewear's Role in an Eye Doctor's Practice

Eyewear operations in eye-care practices deserve the considerable attention they usually get because:

- This is a key step in the eye doctor's prime responsibility to the patient for the visual results and reversal of symptoms the patient expects and deserves.

- This is where the many people who dislike wearing glasses face the unwelcome task of changing their facial appearance with glasses. This is also the reason why many people avoid the eye care from which they would benefit.
- It influences patient loyalty, referrals, and thus patient share.
- It generates important income for the practice.

In the eyewear operation the responsibilities of an eye-care practice are:

- Effective patient care (as in all services)
- Support of regular eye care by helping patients feel good about themselves in eyewear
- Growth of practice and patient share

Eyewear is vital in all three. However, the first point above, "Effective patient care," is so fundamental, so fully acknowledged, and so inherent to the doctor's practice, that it will only be touched on briefly in this chapter. Emphasis would be redundant. The second and third points seem to have had less attention in the eye-care professions, and will thus get attention and emphasis here.

Marketing Eyewear to the Public Today

Outside the eye-care professions, in retail fashion, there is a widely used marketing technique that should probably influence the design and operation of your new eyewear area.

That technique is, "Know your market, and then attract and cater to those people." In an eye-care practice, patients should feel that the eyewear is "for people like me," with a "look I like" (my self-image), and "for doing the things I like to do" (my lifestyle). This focus on patient self-interest should be a theme that is clear to patients in your new eyewear area.

In all but the most economically challenged areas, many shops (not just the fashion boutiques) energetically offer the marketing message, "We respond to *you.*"

Never forget that any eyewear marketing plan must address the powerful motivator, deservedly mentioned so often here, that

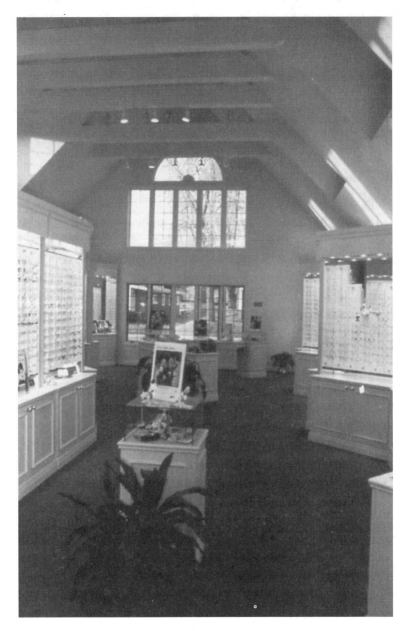

Figure 7–1 The outstanding attractiveness of this setting is powerful evidence supporting the perception of this practice's appreciation of and response to patient sensitivities about glasses. (Reprinted with permission from Drs. Ronald Roelfs and Larry Van Daalen, Waverly, Iowa.)

frequently prevents patients from seeking out eye care: *sensitivity about appearance in glasses*. To market effectively to almost any patient group, your eyewear area should instantly give each patient a convincing perception of your responsiveness to their often deeply felt reluctance or distaste about wearing glasses.

In eyewear, most patient groups (markets) also want continuing attention to traditional patient interests in value, comfort, cost, durability, service, enjoyment of the selection process, etc.

The Vital Unspoken Message

Beyond the necessary perceptions of excellence and dedication to patient care throughout your practice, patients should perceive a compelling message in your eyewear area, from everything seen, including staff. The message is, "You can enjoy your appearance in glasses."

It was only fairly recently that North American eyewear makers appeared to understand that to sell their eyewear, they had to sell ideas.

Garment fashion advertising gets heavy public exposure and is often based on ideas of compelling attractiveness, "the look," "the enviable lifestyle," etc. Close behind, but not dominant, is "buy this item." Their product has strong prominence, but often second to that message of attractiveness. Bear in mind that vendors use the advertising that gets the wanted results.

Eyewear advertisers in North America have adopted this technique. For example, they now emphasize the idea of "enjoying looking good" in eyewear and "having a great time."

Previously, many eyewear ads showed a great-looking model wearing the frame the advertiser wanted you to buy, retouched to be as prominently identifiable as possible. The ad seemed to shout "GLASSES!" Those were the dominant thing—the *only* thing they wanted you to notice on the face (you only saw the face) of an attractive person, and it was a face dominated by glasses.

That kind of ad rubbed peoples' noses in the very look that caused their dislike for wearing glasses. It was rarely effective at suggesting being admired, popular, wanted, having fun, an appealing lifestyle, being up to date, etc.

Eyewear advertising is now much more sophisticated, but the lesson often seems forgotten in the unspoken messages of an eyewear area, where people and eyewear meet. There, public sensitivity about wearing glasses is likely to be strongest because the unwelcome event has arrived—the patient must spend money to get something unwanted but unavoidable.

The Key to Success: Responding to Patient Sensitivity about Appearance in Glasses

In your eyewear area most patients will be at least cheered, often delighted, and sometimes thrilled if they perceive a caring and promising response to their dislike of wearing glasses. That sensitivity to wearing glasses is so deeply felt by the majority of patients, including some who *seem* satisfied, that it merits all the emphasis it gets here. Your perceived response to this remarkably powerful motivator will control or influence most patient's views and decisions about their:

- Level of interest or belief in eyewear as an item of personal attractiveness
- Enjoyment of their own eyewear
- Pleasure over the process of choosing eyewear
- Timing of return for eye care, as motivated by interest in their appearance
- Desire for "special application" eyewear

"Remarkably powerful?" Yes. In fact that's an understatement, as substantiated below.

Here is evidence: It fuels the wealth of the cosmetics industry.

It is the basis for the success of contact lenses, as analyzed earlier. With contact lenses, sensitivity about appearance in glasses has been strong enough to overcome the instinctive aversion to a foreign body on the eye and the resistance to substantial cost, while creating a big demand and a successful industry.

The power of sensitivity about appearance in glasses is even more evident now in the rapidly growing prevalence of expensive corrective surgery on healthy corneas. Despite the cost and risk, many people demand it, even after being cautioned by their doctor.

(The other motivation for this surgery, "convenience and elimination of hassle," seems much less significant.)

How important is personal appearance? Watch someone looking at a top fashion magazine. Some may be turning the pages too fast to be reading. Try interrupting. You will usually find she/he was concentrating. You might be surprised how many people have interest this intense.

Watch the eyes of people looking at a display window. How often are they looking at their own reflection? How often do you do it?

Sensitivity about appearance in glasses crosses gender, age, income, weight, occupation, present appearance, etc. People want to like the way they look.

How is this powerful motivator treated by most of the ophthalmic field? Observe, and you will surely conclude that with few exceptions, this powerful motivator receives inadequate response, or gets lip service or is ignored. But that answer spells *opportunity*.

Because most spectacle wearers *need* glasses and have accepted that verdict, the field has historically and understandably taken the easy route of minimal response to the probable sensitivity of the patient. You likely recognize that most patients make the best of their unwelcome situation, choosing their eyewear in at least an interested, sometimes cheerful, but rarely enthusiastic way. However, most people, yourself included, resent unwanted situations where there is no alternative.

Before contact lenses and LASIK surgery, people needing glasses had no option, although those with a small prescription often went without, as you have surely seen many times. Now patients have these very interesting alternatives to wearing glasses—alternatives that give eyewear some serious competition.

It follows that if the results of eye care and the process of obtaining eyewear were more pleasing and promising, many more patients would come in more often for both. Often, a patient's decision to get needed eye care is swayed or controlled by perceptions, such as what the patient perceives to be your response to his or her sensitivity about wearing glasses.

You will do many things right when you base the design and operation of your eyewear area on responding to this key motivation.

Eyewear as a Fashion Statement

This is an increasingly popular extension of the facial appearance motivation. It needs an effective response in up-to-date eyewear operations.

Patients wanting to make a fashion statement usually have a strong desire to be noticed. Often, they want a particular "group identity" look. Or, they may want far-out eyewear, either from a fashion point of view, or just "to make that statement."

Eyewear area assistants recognize these patients and help them to their goal. "Group identity" and far-out eyewear fashions need space and recognition in your eyewear area.

Targeting *Your* Patients

In almost all locations, a practice serves patients mostly from a local area who usually have a lot in common. This is your patient group, often called your "market."

Your eyewear area should cater to your patient group. Be sure you understand the extent and details of their interest in their appearance, since it will have such a strong impact on your eyewear presentation. That is the marketing technique noted earlier.

Don't jump to what looks to you or your assistants like an obvious answer. Do some research. Ask patients where they buy their fashion items (not work clothes). Observe the cost level of the items in their "casual look." How much care and money has gone into their kind of clothes, etc? A nondescript dress or well-worn overalls may not give a true picture of the wearer's interest in their appearance. This is well known in the fashion and cosmetics fields.

Too often eyewear areas are designed to present eyewear divided only into traditional patient categories: "men's, women's, children's," and perhaps, "full time, reading, safety, sun wear, etc." Patients may see this as the same old setup. It could reduce their loyalty to you, particularly if someplace more promising is available, even at higher cost or an inconvenient distance. Or they might come in as infrequently as possible. Or, after deciding, "There's nothing really interesting here," they might go elsewhere to try some advertised lower prices.

For your patients, a visit to your eyewear area should be a welcome *event*, not just another visit to a place with those masses

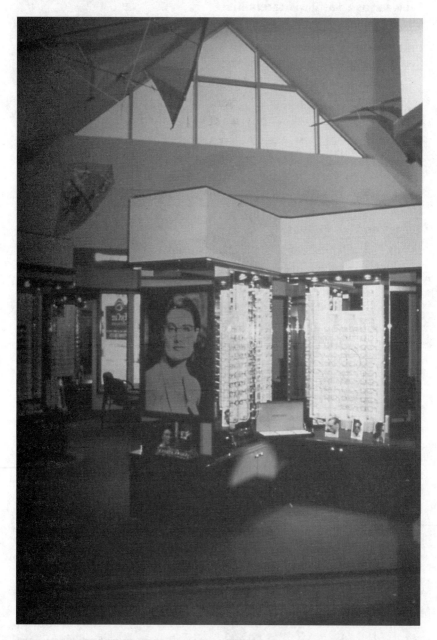

Figure 7–2 The vaulted ceiling, natural light, and use of mass and feature display make this strong functionally and in the key area of perceptions. (Reprinted with permission of the American Optometric Association. *AOA News*, October 1998; 10D.)

of frames. Patients who perceive you as keeping up with modern trends for them feel better about using your services, giving you a steadily increasing patient share in your area.

How is this done? An example may help. For young urban professionals (an upscale suburb or bedroom community) you could:

- Decorate their area to be bright and colorful
- Stress value
- Expand the kids' section
- Have an outdoors section with rugged eyewear for climbing, hiking, ski goggle inserts, oversized ski goggles to fit over eyewear, etc.
- Have men's and women's high-fashion sections, including the latest "business look"
- Have a section with styles for those who want to "make a statement"

For senior patients use a well-lighted area, but with less flash than above, comfortable chairs with arms, and of course, suitable eyewear (for fashion and their lifestyle).

Development of this eyewear area is one of the challenges to be entrusted to your designer—someone experienced in your profession's facilities *and* retail fashion stores, or with access to that experienced advice. Also, get guidance from the better frame reps, and from observing how the more successful local non-eyewear fashion stores respond to this market.

Patient Recognition of Superiority

Plan and design your eyewear area to be instantly perceived as superior. The staff, decor, lighting, kinds of displays, recognized signature styles, and much more—all should seem to patients and visitors to be the best they have seen.

Patients want the reassuring perception of your frame area's superiority, as reassurance that they have done the right thing in coming to you despite the constant advertising by discounters claiming or implying, "We Sell You the Same Thing for Less."

Location of Your Eyewear Area

Choose the location (and design) of your eyewear area in your practice to complement your practice style *and* make a statement about your entire operation.

It is tempting to locate it as the first and most impressive thing seen on entering the practice, or to locate it in separate space beside your practice, perhaps with its own name, entrance, and signage. These ideas tend to be based on meeting competition.

But consider the drawbacks. Located at your entrance, your eyewear area can tend to dominate your practice and thus be perceived as your main mission. This evidence can too easily blur the patient's perception of whether you are a doctor or a merchant.

With your eyewear operation in a separate location, you risk the unwanted patient perception that you have little or no involvement in their satisfaction from the total eye-care service they need. Compare this to being perceived as fully, proudly, and happily responsible for all aspects of their eye care—a perception that is supported by having your eyewear area and other dispensing functions within your practice.

You can have a lot at stake here. For credibility as a health-care operation, your practice needs to be correctly perceived as run by a *doctor* dedicated to the care that a patient expects and wants—from clinical services and, almost as important, from superior, patient-care eyewear services. That perception is why so many people prefer to receive all aspects of their eye care from a trusted and respected eye doctor. That perception and patient pleasure with eyewear choice will give your practice vital competitive strength.

Designing to combine two such different functions as the clinical and eyewear sides of an eye-care practice, while sustaining convincing perceptions of your status as a doctor, calls for both skill and experience, often in some combination from you and a suitably qualified designer.

Your eyewear area should rarely be the most impressive thing seen *on entering your office*. Patient and public perceptions of the primacy of clinical diagnostic and treatment services in your office must start with noticeable, supporting evidence at its front end, and then in the area of your grouped clinical services. At the same time, your valid need to win perceptions of clinical priority should never result in an eyewear operation that is less than the best it can be.

Your eyewear area's location contributes to those patient perceptions. It can be located so its attractiveness is seen from the front or the clinical services access route. Although it needs to be the finest your designer can do, it shouldn't be perceived as your dominant function.

It merits repeating: your patients will be most comfortable when they perceive you as their doctor.

An Alternative Outside Your Practice: The Licensed Dispensing Optician

The time-honored alternative method of supplying dispensing services to the public is of course through an independent licensed dispensing optician. A good one can do this very well. The comparative merits of this alternative is not the subject of this book, but will undoubtedly be hotly contested long into the future.

Size and Capacity

The size of the eyewear area in an eye-care practice is usually a compromise among its space needs for other practice functions, and the cost. There will be two key criteria:

1. The eyewear area must be big enough for consistent high standards when operating at forecasted capacity.
2. It must be big enough to impress patients and thus help win their confidence and enthusiasm.

To estimate the number of patients to be served at one time, forecast the following:

1. The number of patients per hour discharged from the diagnostic side
2. The percentage of those patients who will use your eyewear area

3. The average time required per patient for eyewear selection

Assuming that each patient for eyewear will be served by an eyewear assistant, you will need one assistant and one eyewear choice station per patient anticipated there during normal operation. The area should be big enough for the stations to handle the patient numbers after at least five years' growth.

Because patient time choosing eyewear (and lenses if done there) varies, the eyewear area will sometimes be too small (not enough stations). At other times it may be "slow" or empty.

When patient numbers increase but assistant stations can't, patients will have to wait more often, and for a longer time. When that happens, those waiting could be invited to browse unescorted, even if you prefer that all processes of eyewear selection should always be assistant guided. If browsing is feasible, some or all of the eyewear area would have to be set up for it.

If the initial design reveals that the eyewear area is going to be too small, you may have strong evidence that your total facility isn't big enough. If you are committed to the place by a lease or ownership, you will want some way of getting a larger eyewear area, while minimizing the damage of taking space from other practice functions. Because your eyewear area is so important to your patients and your practice, ask your designer to help you find practice functions that could be accommodated in smaller spaces, combined, or perhaps even omitted.

When Speed Is Needed

Time is important to most patients, very important to others. Some of the latter are patients who haven't found time for eye care for far too long. Others may be regular patients with a tight schedule. Their need for speed is often known in the practice (probably noted on their clinical record), or if this is their first visit, recognized by an assistant or the doctor.

Flag this patient's record as a "don't-delay" person. I'm not suggesting that such a patient go ahead of others, as this can raise justifiable anger in those bypassed. But all along the path of a don't-delay patient, steps should be taken and organization should be in place that will speed up service.

Try to have all eyewear stations self-contained as fully equipped units, designed and organized both for normal operating efficiency and to provide speed when wanted.

Put these eyewear orders in the usual red job trays, but always label them conspicuously with an honest deadline rather than the less meaningful words "Rush" and "Super Rush." Seeing the deadline, lab staff will know when this job is needed.

Assistant-Guided Selection Versus Browsing

You may decide that both assistant-guided selection and browsing are needed in your practice, even if you favor only one. Of course, either or both must be well organized.

Usually an assistant, or perhaps the doctor escorts the patient to your eyewear area. If the escorting person is not one of the eyewear staff, the patient will be welcomed at "eyewear" by one of the assistants there.

This seems a good place to emphasize that the term "eyewear assistant" is a generalization. Most practices will benefit greatly from having dispensing functions performed by a good, licensed dispensing optician whose knowledge will be valuable to the patient and thus the practice.

At the entrance to the eyewear area, the decor, the staff, and an impressive, informative array of feature displays should win perceptions of fashion.

Feature displays are proven techniques for informing patients in ways they tend to like. Backlighted photo transparencies showing attractive eyewear on appealing people doing interesting things are particularly effective. Feature displays silently answer the patient's often eager questions about fashion: "What's new in signature eyewear? What are the trends?", etc. These stories and impressions can give the patient a positive frame of mind.

Some patients will want to do what they call "look around" (introductory browsing), which is one way of starting eyewear selection. Mostly, such browsing lasts for only a short time. Although browsing generally is at its best when guided by an eyewear assistant, some patients will prefer to be unaccompanied. Some (not many) firmly prefer to only select eyewear by browsing, either with an assistant or unescorted. However, even they know they must finally be served by an assistant. (If patients are unescorted browsers only because they are waiting for a free assistant, isn't that revealing your need for more staff, and/or greater eyewear area capacity?)

Other patients will prefer going directly to "one-on-one" selection. Many people with strong sensitivity about their appearance in glasses are unhappy selecting eyewear by browsing. They often prefer to put their confidence in an assistant whose appearance and manner suggest skill and high qualifications.

One-on-one presentation has proven itself in fashion, cosmetics, and jewelry shops, operations that often deal with strong sensitivity about appearance. In first-rate retail stores, most cosmetics and better fashion items are actively presented by trained people, but sometimes are racked for self-service.

Most ophthalmic consultants I have met or heard advocate one-on-one eyewear presentation. In their view and mine it is the winner in satisfying most patients, partly because good eyewear assistants recognize and respond to patient sensitivities, interests, and self-image. Talented, well-trained, informed assistants usually make the process and result of eyewear selection as pleasant as it can be, depending on the patient's level of aversion to glasses.

Some doctors want patients to browse (or be free to do so) during dilation. If available, assistants should work with these patients. If not, the patient can still, through exposure to feature displays, have an interesting, perhaps stimulating time being informed about eyewear. Incidentally, in a large practice these patients should probably be given a pager to alert them when it's time for them to return to the exam room.

Your decision whether to organize your eyewear area and displays for selection that is assistant guided only, browsing only, or both will usually depend on:

- Which, in your view, will function most effectively for patients and practice
- The image you want for your eyewear operation
- The demographics of your patient group
- Matching competition (not as important as you might expect)

- The views of your more experienced eyewear staff
- Space availability, etc.

Even if you favor one-on-one selection, you will probably feel the need to accommodate some browsers, both accompanied and unescorted.

Crowding

The relatives, friends, etc., who are sometimes with patients can crowd selection stations and/or the browsing area. Unless this happens too frequently or your eyewear area is too small, this could be an opportunity, not a problem, as some guests are potential patients. Skilled assistants can usually handle this, and win admiration from both patient and guest. If there is no room for guests at a selection station or the browsing area, try to seat them elsewhere in the eyewear area. As a last choice, use the nearby internal waiting.

Seated or Standing Selection

When a patient and assistant are both comfortably seated, eyewear selection more often wins patient satisfaction, or (better still) pleasure, or (best) enthusiasm. When patients are seated and thus more likely to be relaxed, they usually find it easier to concentrate on the process and desired result, and to appreciate the ideas and suggestions being presented to them. Seated selection is the norm in the eyewear operations of most eye doctors, except perhaps the extremely busy ones, where minimum time is the top priority.

Seated eyewear selection helps staff get accurate measurements of vertical heights for optical centers, multifocal segments, and progressive lens reference points, because the assistant's line of sight to the patient's eyes is then close to horizontal. When the patient and assistant differ significantly in height, an assistant's chair with an easy-to-use vertical adjustment will help (also needed at eyewear delivery services.)

If there is room in the eyewear area, all seated stations should have two chairs, one each for the patient and a guest. To avoid crowding, the chairs should obviously not be large. If your eyewear area is carpeted (highly probable), chairs might have carpet casters for mobility. These chairs could also be an element of decor that contributes to perceptions of fashion. They could also be distinctively masculine or feminine as a clue to help identify these areas (overcoming any temptation to use signs).

In very busy practices, some eyewear assistants prefer standing eyewear selection. They say that it usually takes less time than seated, and is less tiring because it doesn't involve constantly sitting down and standing up. They prefer remaining on their feet, and the welcome activity of walking around. If standing eyewear selection is preferred by you and your staff, remember that this could be unwelcome to a lot of patients, so quite a few seated stations will still be needed for those patients who want or need to be seated.

Even with patients who prefer to stand, eyewear selection that starts stand-up (perhaps done entirely by browsing) usually ends seated. However, in that very busy, browsing-style, stand-up eyewear operation, there may be no seated station open, so selection will then have to be concluded standing.

Eyewear stations with standing assistants could be equipped with patient bar stools so they can sit, or support their rear end. Bar stools could be a hit with young adult and teen patients, and cheerfully accepted by many others. But they are not recommended for patients who don't like them, or are unsteady on their feet, who would need a station with normal seating. Avoid bar stools on casters, as they could move away when a patient leans on or climbs onto the seat.

When all eyewear assistants are occupied, some newly arrived patients and those that have finished browsing will be kept waiting. If this happens often, you may be tempted to use "two-on-one" selection stations, where two patients are served at the same time by the same assistant. These stations are usually "L" shaped with the patients outside the arms of the "L" and the assistant inside. The assistant turns ninety degrees to serve the other patient.

This two-on-one operation risks the happiness of patients wanting undivided attention (a reasonable desire), or who realize that they are in fact still waiting, since when one patient gets attention, the other mostly waits. While both are seated at the station, they each want and need to feel that they are being served. Also, reduced privacy could lead to patient dissatisfaction, or assistant difficulty in sensitive situations.

Your decision on seated, standing, or combined eyewear selection will as usual depend on the space limitations and other problems in your eyewear area, and your view of what will be best, first for your patients, and then for the practice.

How Many Frames?

Eye doctors and assistants might often answer, "Patients should perceive *a lot*." That perceptual target has merit, but only to the extent that there shouldn't seem to be too few.

Should "number of frames" be an issue in an eye doctor's eyewear operations? Perhaps the answer is "Sometimes, but rarely." Your eyewear operation should usually be able to win patient perceptions far more effective than "a lot of frames," such as:

- "This is my kind of place."
- "I'm starting to feel better about wearing glasses."
- "This place is filled with interesting stuff and ideas."
- "I wonder if I could like how I look in glasses?"
- "This place sure has changed from the way it used to be."
- "This might be fun."
- "I wonder if I should have a pair of those for my _____ (hobby, sport, etc.)."
- "That picture looks great—wonder how I'd look in that frame?"

Few of these perceptions are likely to be won by displays that inadvertently or deliberately emphasize a large number of frames.

As discussed in the sections that follow, if your displays earn the positive and even enthusiastic perceptions just listed, those perceptions will to a considerable extent result from effective feature presentations.

Often, and justifiably, your thinking on this point will be influenced by local competition, particularly a competitor who aggressively and constantly advertises thousands of frames. Try not to get hung up on matching such a competitor. Choose a better, different way to compete. This is a time-honored and sound strategy.

When your displays are truly interesting, intriguing, promising, compelling (you name the positive impact), causing patients to experience pleasant feelings of anticipation, hope, comfort, and curiosity, few of them will consider whether you have a lot, enough, or too few frames. Eyewear numbers will rarely register.

However, some patients *expect* to see a lot of frames. That expectation could seem an important issue. This should occur infrequently, because even that patient's interest in "a lot" will often be outweighed by the appeal of your promising, exciting frames and ideas.

If winning the perception of "a lot of eyewear" is important to you, bear in mind that the perception isn't based on numbers alone. The perception of "a lot" will tend to occur when your frame quantity is above a "too small" minimum, reasonable for the size of your practice, *and when all eyewear displays are filled* (no obvious empty slots), including feature displays that show frames along with compelling photographs and information.

Patient perceptions about numbers of displayed eyewear can be surprising. Patients in a fine new eyewear area, with no more or even fewer frames than before, surprise eye doctors with the comment, "You have so many more frames now." Perception is reality to the viewer.

After considering all factors, you must tell your designer how many frames you want on display so that she/he can design or specify display fixtures to hold that approximate total.

In an established practice, the number of frames on display will often be influenced and sometimes controlled by:

- The size of the practice
- The size (display capacity) of the eyewear area
- The demographics (including lifestyles) of the majority of your patient group
- Your mix (if any) of mass and feature display
- The cost of inventory
- Your convictions on the best way for you to do very well despite the competition

Your consultant/designer and/or your marketing/management consultant should be able to help you choose how many frames to display in your eyewear area. See Chapter 10 for ideas on the number of frames to display in a startup practice.

Display Objectives

The range of objectives of displays throughout your practices includes

- To inform patients about the care of their eyes and vision
- To inform patients about your materials, services, policies, etc.
- To reduce their anxieties
- To win their pleasure, enthusiasm, and loyalty.

Displays that do this will help your practice grow faster and surpass competition more easily.

Eyewear displays are usually the main interface between eyewear and patients. The right patient responses to eyewear displays should make it easy for them to choose frames, and often reduce

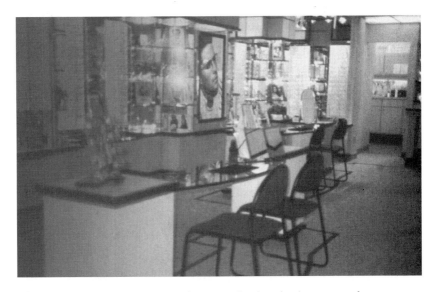

Figure 7–3 Eyewear area, made attractive by spaciousness, glass counters, feature and mass displays, and no sense of crowding delivers both an effective operation and the right perceptions. (Reprinted with permission from Dr. Tom McWilliams, Prairie Du Chien, Wisconsin.)

concerns about wearing glasses, or convert some concerns to confidence. To make this powerful contribution to your eyewear selection, your frame displays must be highly impressive, second only to the work of your eyewear assistants. Figures 7-3 and 7-4 show ways this can be done.

Your displays (not just those in your eyewear area) should help make patients feel:

- That you are (perhaps unexpectedly) responsive and sympathetic to their sensitivity about their appearance in glasses
- That their other interests and wishes are recognized and catered to
- That this is a patient-friendly place
- That your practice offers excellent technical lens knowledge and skill (although these displays don't belong in the eyewear area—see Chapter 8)
- That your practice is sophisticated and up-to-date—they won't do better elsewhere

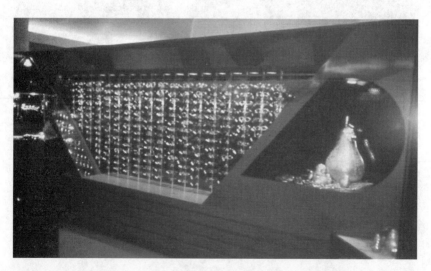

Figure 7–4 Dramatic mass display shows how strong this technique can be, particularly when combined with the compelling adjacent feature displays. (Reprinted with permission from Dr. Arnold Stokol, Richardson, Texas.)

and much more. (See the section later in this chapter, "Perceptions and Messages.")

Traditionally and at this time, the winning of perceptual objectives and the delivery of information about current fashions falls almost entirely on the shoulders of eyewear staff. They usually do an outstanding job, mostly with only modest help from displays (visual evidence). Even with the best displays, your staff will be the main contributors to the success of your eyewear area. But the perceptions delivered by appropriate displays will give them a powerful ally, to the benefit of both your patients and practice.

Mass Display

Has it outlived its usefulness? Good points can be advanced in support of both the "Yes" and the "No" answers.

The main arguments in favor of mass display are:

1. It is used in many successful eyewear operations and has a long track record.
2. It can be done in an elegant, impressive way that wins good perceptions.
3. It invites and suits unescorted browsing, which means you need fewer staff.
4. It is comfortably familiar to many people both in eyewear and retailing, so they feel at ease going in and trying on eyewear.
5. It instantly suggests "A lot of eyewear, no shortage of choice."
6. It is relatively easy to set up as a display and needs little creative talent.

The main arguments against mass display are:

1. It fails or is relatively ineffective at informing people about:
   - Your caring, promising response to their negative feelings about their appearance in glasses
   - Availability of eyewear that meets their lifestyle interests
   - What's new in numerous leading signature lines

- Current fashion trends (the "look," the "in" color, etc.)
- The superior and clearly distinctive nature of your eyewear operation
2. Mass is less effective than feature displays in marketing your eyewear operation (e.g., winning a range of patient perceptions or delivering a variety of information).
3. Mass display is the look of the discount dispensary.
4. It is not a fashion-based method of display. Mass displays look more like racks of goods than a fashion presentation.
5. It is uninterestingly familiar. Display techniques that are notably more current would usually generate more patient interest and positive responses.

The mass display concept seems to be: If 500 frames are impressive, 1,000 must be twice as impressive, and 2,000 would be even better (until someone advertises 3,000).

Although mass display is used widely today, it invites criticism because as presently used, it yields shrinking benefits to the patient and the private eye-care practice, as discussed below.

Here are some claimed mass display advantages, with the observable drawbacks of each:

Massive Choice That Will Satisfy Most Patients

This is losing its appeal. The unexpected popularity of signature styles has shown the ophthalmic field that surprising numbers of people can feel better about their appearance in glasses. Their numbers reveal the power of negative public feelings about eyewear and the power of an idea other than "massive choice."

The move from massive choice toward the entirely different, much more promising attraction of signature styles is creating unprecedented growth in the eye-care/eyewear fields. Yet many eyewear providers, while enjoying the success of signature eyewear, continue to concentrate their displays in mass presentation that offers little convincing evidence that this is a fashion place.

By itself, mass display is the look of an outlet, a place where price tends to be the main attraction—a marketing technique that makes it unclear whether your main appeal is fashion or price.

Many patients will reject the idea that a mass-display, price-based operation is a true fashion source.

Consider the phrase "fashion source." Some people feel better about themselves when they call a mass-display, discount clothing outlet a "fashion source," usually because it is where *they* shop. But others (the growing number of better informed people) will often prefer the real thing and choose to afford it, as long as identical items aren't being offered for less elsewhere.

Factors other than price, when presented in understandable, believable ways, are likely to motivate the choices of many who are sensitive about their appearance in glasses. But mass display will succeed by default when no inviting alternative is offered. As noted above, mass display operations usually draw people to whom price is dominant, and others who don't know or believe that any better alternative exists.

To tap the power of fashion, a place must look the part, with evidence successfully presenting the message, "This place looks promising. Maybe wearing glasses could be interesting, not a 'drag,' not just a necessity."

Talk this over with your marketing advisers and those in the design field before making your final decisions about the design of your eyewear area.

Mass Display Perceived as Up-to-Date

This is unlikely since, in other fashion fields better display techniques exist and flourish. Your patients will see these other display techniques in an increasing number of nonoptical places, some of which they may patronize.

Some people neglect their eye care because they are attracted to spend their money on other, more appealing things, particularly other fashion items. Updating eyewear display methods seems to be a neglected point in marketing your field *in competition with other fashion fields*.

Perhaps worse for you as a doctor is the public perception that mass display is the look of the optical discounter (and some chains). You need to be instantly perceived as at least different, preferably superior.

In other fashion fields, display techniques are constantly improved by display designers, at the insistent demand of retailers whose display designs must be cutting edge because the retailer's success depends on it, and their competitors are or will be doing it.

Despite its decline, some mass display may be needed to accommodate browsing but usually only in part of your eyewear area. But now that signature eyewear has arrived, the field needs more of the innovation seen in other fields: new, more attractive and fashion oriented displays, typified by feature displays.

Combining Mass and Feature Displays

Mass display eyewear presentation will usually need to include feature displays.

In combining mass and feature displays, aim to respond to the broad and the specific interests of your patients. Think of your eyewear displays as many of your patients would.

How will your eyewear area be perceived by male and female patients of various ages young, teen, a little older, or elderly? Will they know where to look? Does it look uninteresting? Will it all seem patient friendly?

What follows are some mostly familiar alternative ways of setting up combined mass and feature display eyewear areas, each with its design needs, its benefits, and its drawbacks. In each of these there will be gains and losses for patients and practice, and there are no clearly obvious choices.

Traditional Categories of Men, Women, Children, Unisex, Teens

Here, people will identify the eyewear divisions for gender and age from signs, decor, atmosphere (perhaps lighting), props, and (most important) feature displays. Or, staff will tell them. Signs for this purpose will reduce your eyewear area's credibility as a fashion source. When signs alone indicate the "Men's" or "Women's" areas, patients perceive that you:

- Are unwilling to cater to women as women and men as men
- Are insensitive to the idea
- Don't know how to do it without signs

A sign might be needed for the big eyewear segment Unisex. Or you could show feature display photographs of men and women both clearly wearing the same Unisex eyewear.

Children's is easier, as the familiar props (a kind of feature display) are almost always understood instantly by children and parents.

Teens often want their group's look-alike appearance, but with clearly different, distinctive eyewear and in an atmosphere both instantly and unmistakably seen to be as different as possible from anything that would attract their parents or their subteen siblings. That's a designer's challenge.

And, within each traditional category, some patients will want to know, "Where are the most popular frames? Where are the things I'd want to see? Where do I start looking?" Feature displays can help answer their questions.

Organize by Lifestyle

Because this kind of marketing is so popular (for the results it gets) in the highly competitive world of fashion marketing, it should be familiar and reassuring to many of your patients and deserves to be a leading contender in the successful development of display in your new or reworked eyewear area.

Lifestyle marketing in eyewear is made-to-order for feature displays, and difficult to handle with mass display alone. Your designer and/or vendor should be able to help you organize some feature displays into effective, dynamic lifestyle eyewear stories.

Organize by Eyewear Popularity

This has been used for years by experienced eyewear area managers and staff who find that it saves them time and effort. It is also the basis of the time-honored staff practice of putting their favorite styles in the best display positions.

Is it a good idea? To a considerable extent the answer is "Yes." Popular styles are in demand, usually because they have a lot going for them. This is why the staff favors them, although the reverse is also true: staff can influence which styles become popular. It looks like a "win–win" situation because popular eyewear usually achieves patient satisfaction or even delight, while also speeding the selection process, valuable in busy (and probably almost all) eyewear areas.

A word of caution is needed here. Many patients will appreciate seeing feature displays showing new eyewear styles that are promising but not yet popular. That exposure informs patients about what is now possible, and you have the advantage that they see it in your office, not someplace else. Admittedly, this could slow the selection process, but it will interest many patients. Even if they don't choose one of these new styles, seeing them could win a return visit.

Organize by Cost to the Patient

Some patients in some practices will like this. Emphasis on price/cost can seem a good idea, and sometimes will be. But strong emphasis on price could invite problems. Price-based operations are widespread in your field. Some are successful, some not. Their market share will of course depend in part on their operation and the location or region they're in. For you to succeed in competing with a strong low-price operation, your private practice will probably need to be instantly perceived as different and better in ways that appeal locally, probably including a totally distinctive eyewear area and marketing program.

It is a complex subject. Here are a few points for your consideration.

The media deluge of price advertising ("the same for less") has over the years sensitized many people to the lure and the doubts associated with price. Price affects most of us. But the volume and nature of price advertising has created a number of people (particularly the better informed and educated) who tend to have less faith in advertised claims. Value ("what I get for my money"), rather than price alone, now seems a bigger influence on today's better-informed patient.

Throughout a practice, helping patients recognize real rather than claimed value benefits both sides. Value will be most believable when reliable, consistent evidence fully supports it. Feature displays and demonstrations by staff are needed.

Talking to the patient about value (explanations, details, etc.) can be helpful, but also risky. Remember the Shakespeare quotation, "Methinks he doth protest too much." Consider how you respond when a person you haven't doubted keeps saying, "I'm telling you the truth."

Organizing eyewear displays by price offers some gain, but mainly with those relatively few patients who make their choice on cost alone. Your experience probably tells you that although price is often a factor, most patients choose on a single, subjective point: "I like it," or "I don't like it:" Even in a discount operation, "Do I like it?" is the basis of choice far more than price.

Enlighten patients about value by the most effective and efficient means available. Until they're shown, most patients usually can't recognize which eyewear is excellent, mediocre, and inferior. The value of newness will sometimes be even more difficult to establish.

Awareness of value might be supported by having each value level in its own part of your eyewear area, using decor, feature displays, and props supporting the value of the items.

There could be good reasons to organize by price, but an alternative that *includes* price might be better, as with the following three groupings based on the dominant interest of the patient:

- Cost dominated (smallest group?)
- Fashion dominated (mid-sized group?)
- Cost and fashion dominated (largest group?)

This way the emphasis in the last two groups would be on patient benefits, attractive for reasons other than cost alone. Within each group, you could have sections that present some of the other areas of patient interest that are under discussion here (men's, women's, kids', teens', unisex, lifestyle, etc.). Yes, it's getting too complicated to be workable.

Finally, should the eyewear be priced in an eyewear area that is organized by cost?

Organize by Fashion, Particularly Signature Styles

The appeal of signature styles has led to impressive new public acceptance of eyewear. This has shown that powerful enough *fashion* images can inspire public interest in and even enthusiasm for eyewear.

Eyewear areas focused on fashion should display signature frames prominently, in highly attractive, specialized feature displays (discussed later). Because so many people find signature and other special eyewear interesting, their displays stand a better chance of being powerfully effective (noticed, understood, and believed), particularly when well conceived and executed. One doctor reported having patients order designer frames with plano lenses, which they wanted to wear for their business look. You probably know similar stories.

Organize by Patient Demographics

Will patients be most satisfied with your eyewear operation when your display techniques and frames are tied to local demographics? The answer seems to be, "Yes, but it will be better if the fashion range is broader than suggested by the demographics." Remember that in the present era of TV, travel, the Internet, etc., fashion tastes are more broad ranging. Past regional, urban versus rural, and even affluent versus less affluent demographic differences are fading.

Still, you wouldn't offer the same eyewear in an economically challenged area as in an upscale suburb. The fashion trends would be similar, but the price point would be lower.

Most citizens in lower income areas want to look good, feel good about themselves, and be catered to like people who are better off. This should be reflected in the eyewear area decor and displays. As you know, these patients usually want (need) these results but at a lower cost, and yet are often experienced enough to have little or no confidence in the very lowest priced aggressively advertised items that their circumstances may force them to choose.

You will undoubtedly respond to patient demographics (local patient preferences in style and performance) by shifting the fashion and cost range of your eyewear up or down. But be careful. You already know that patient choice can be unpredictable in fashion level, cost, etc.

The level of eyewear displayed or shown to a patient can depend on your assistant's comfort in inventorying and offering it. If the assistant is from a less affluent area (perhaps where the practice is located), a patient won't be shown something better that they would like to see because it does or could interest them, perhaps because they saw it being worn or in a shop window. Either the frame was rejected for display or, if there, it wasn't shown because the assistant was sure patients would feel it is too expensive—which could of course be right, but shouldn't be a generalized assumption.

Regardless of demographics or price point, always use impressive displays so all patients will be attracted by your high standards, and will feel catered to (regardless of their economic status). Even in low-income areas, handsome display fixtures will rarely frighten patients away from your eyewear area, because most will recognize and appreciate that you are treating each of them as someone important (as they are).

Other Needs in Display Organization

You may want an acceptable, effective way of "moving" certain frames. The "On Sale" display (discussed later under "signs") should take care of this, or you could have on-sale eyewear in attractive display trays in a cabinet to be shown to patients who have been recognized as wanting lowest cost.

You may want some displays to answer the question, "What's new?"—another job done best by feature displays. Some patients who see or are shown that you have a regularly updated "what's new" display, which they are invited to see on a curiosity-satisfying, drop-in basis, will be delighted and impressed with this new, unusual (for eyewear operations) service.

Two Overlooked, Time-Honored Approaches

In the eyewear field, one of the biggest style application factors is ignored or treated casually. Yet it is a time-honored, central concept in much of the fashion field, namely the differences between the sexes.

For how many hundreds of years have there been different shops for men's and women's clothing? In an eyewear area, these categories may be separated, but these groupings are sometimes hard to distinguish because the look of each area doesn't change to identify and convey a credible sense of catering to male and female interests.

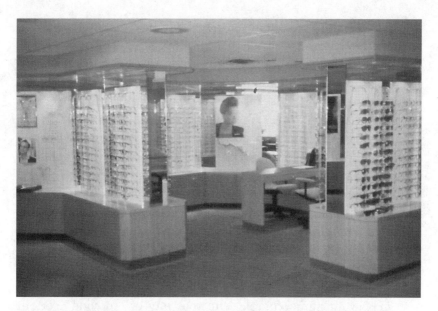

Figure 7–5 Women are catered to here, with a separate area, easily identified by large, appropriate backlighted photographs. (Reprinted with permission from Dr. Gene Zackowski, Creston, British Columbia.)

Women's shops that carry only formal wear, only business outfits, only casual wear, etc., abound and are widely accepted as familiar sources of excellence in their category of fashion and performance. Also, department stores and other shops that offer more than one style category usually present each division (department?) distinctively, to be attractive and thus effective for its purpose and to be easily identified.

Separate fashion application is a totally familiar, highly accepted theme—except in eyewear. Here, this concept, if presented at all, may be served by no more than one or two feature displays or signs. Why shouldn't this established fashion concept be followed in eyewear?

One male eyewear assistant in a large practice complained of the scarcity of male-oriented displays. How many male patients sense or notice this?

This widely appreciated approach deserves more consideration than it usually gets.

Pricing All Displayed Eyewear

Should eyewear be priced in all systems? There are good reasons to show prices even though in almost all practices selection by price alone is small ranging down to insignificant.

Obviously, the top reason for showing prices is that it permits patients to use this comfortable and familiar system of budgeting by comparing prices. Most patients, while choosing on the basis of "Do I like it?" want to see the price so they can react silently, which for them means privately. This is their everyday way of managing their spending.

Open pricing also suggests that you have open ways, which please many patients and build their confidence.

Capable, knowledgeable eyewear assistants can skillfully clarify the value involved by presenting the reasons for a price. This will often help the patient decide and feel comfortable about spending what is needed to go ahead with "the frame I like."

The potential risks are of course a price higher than competition and/or a patient's, or your market's perception that in general your prices are too high. However, you will also face this (although probably less often) when prices are quoted rather than on the item.

Change Alone Can Help You

Be open to change in eyewear groupings, locations, and methods of display. Change alone is stimulating for both patients and staff. Positive patient responses to attractive, noticeable change (perhaps in feature displays) offers your practice the additional, perhaps unexpected reward of a stronger image.

Conclusions

You will recognize that mass display of eyewear is a mixed blessing. By its nature, mass display alone doesn't do enough to encourage and/or respond effectively to patient interest in:

- Fashion application in eyewear
- Signature fashions
- "Lifestyle" eyewear
- Information and ideas

• Perceptions that could build patient confidence and please them

If mass display is the one you want, be sure it is supported generously by the versatility and strengths of skillfully applied feature displays.

Among the ideas presented here, some may seem too "far out." Possibly they are. But an innovative doctor could be building patient perceptions that she/he is a leader, not a follower.

Feature Display

The absence of feature display severely slowed public acceptance of eyewear as "fashion" in the early days of fashion choice. In eyewear, feature display still has a long way to go.

Historically eyewear feature displays were almost always only in windows. The better ones were frequently done by someone felt to be an expert (on staff, or hired for the purpose). In those days few owners of eyewear operations were aware of the feature display concept or thought of using suitably talented people to do this creative work.

In the quite recent but still bad old days, before doctors and the public woke up to the possibilities for public interest in eyewear, feature display was still absent or used sparingly in a half-hearted way. How many ophthalmic practitioners predicted the positive public response to signature eyewear?

Signature eyewear presentation is an exercise in feature display. Small, clearly identified groups of effectively identified "special" eyewear are shown. Each should be supported by a photograph and props that are often unrelated fashion products with the same designer or celebrity brand.

Many eyewear operation managers seemed uncertain how to present signature frames, particularly in a mass display format. They recognized their need for signature styles, obtained them, and then had to find an effective way and an adequate place to display them.

Fashion product feature displays can be seen in most, if not all, other fashion fields. Men's and women's shops use them in windows and throughout the interior to:

- Create the appropriate atmosphere
- Announce their responsiveness to the market they serve and wish to attract
- Introduce and win support for an idea or item
- Show how attractive, interesting, loveable, successful, athletic, etc., a person can be, wearing or using this product

In a mall's high pedestrian traffic, fashion and non-fashion shops often count on feature displays at their entrance to be "stoppers," getting attention among passersby and then attracting some to enter (a challenging assignment).

In the eyewear field, the extensive use of feature display has the added advantage that it is still relatively new. Patients will rarely have encountered the eyewear ideas and stories you will be presenting this way. Those ideas will inform the patients and often win valuable perceptions of your eyewear operation.

These displays will use their recognizably novel technique to identify and emphasize patient benefits. You should expect your feature displays to:

- Tell of appealing attractiveness and lifestyle enhancement
- Make your patient group feel recognized, comfortable, and confident
- Present the features of special eyewear, the attractiveness and reasons for sunglasses, the advantages of accessories, the stories supporting value, and much more

As noted repeatedly here, your feature displays should put you ahead of much of your competition.

Feature Display to Inform Patients

Eyewear area feature displays should be based on the interests of patients. The displays should give them both specific and general information, mainly to answer one question: "What can these new trends in eyewear really do for *me*?"

Feature displays should therefore respond to patient interest in:

1. What's new in signature frames?
2. What is popular now?

3. What are the fashion trends?
4. What is "the look" at this time?
5. What are the "in" colors?
6. What is there here for me (my kind of person) with my lifestyle, my interests?
7. What is "far out," that I will rarely if ever see on other people?

Choosing the patient questions and interests to address in your feature displays will be a demanding opportunity. You will rarely have room for enough displays to meet all patient interests. But it's a nice problem, and a nice change, to be choosing each month which *positive* patient interests you will respond to (interests that are often unstated and even unrecognized by the patient).

Without feature displays to inform patients and win the right perceptions, the entire burden falls on your eyewear area staff, who undoubtedly do it well. But do you and they feel that this repetitive, time-consuming job is the best use of their skills and experience?

Even with notable feature displays, your assistants will continue to be occupied, often fully, with the challenging and often lengthy job of deciding what a patient needs (or wants?) and then responding to both the individuality of that patient, and his/her expressed and/or unvoiced wishes in eyewear.

I believe most eyewear area staff would like the support of a full range of informative feature displays, so the patients they work with will have ideas about the eyewear that interests them (and will often have a more positive attitude). The shared task of informing patients will require feature displays readily available for patient viewing in much or all of your eyewear area.

As noted above, you probably won't ever have enough feature displays. This introduces the need for a program of display updating, offering you the valuable opportunity to attract visits by some patients. Think how much a drop-in visit to your eyewear area could appeal to a segment of your patients when they know you will have specific displays that are regularly and often renewed (preferably on a timetable). By occasionally dropping in, as invited by the eyewear assistants, these more fashion-motivated patients see the latest in eyewear that could be fascinating to them.

The concept of fashion-inspired drop-in visits may be hard for you and your staff to accept, as you are presumably all busy enough already, and in this instance the visit would not necessarily result in immediate income. Ask yourself, should you and your eyewear assistants oppose fashion-motivated drop-in visits because you want only patients who have a prescription to be filled?

The items and information in your feature displays should respond to the wide range of your patients' interests and needs. The stories should go far beyond the present worthy emphasis on attractiveness in glasses. Feature displays for men and women should identify fashion and activity-related eyewear suitable within your patient group (market) for the following applications:

- Business
- Casual wear
- Hobbies
- Athletic pursuits
- Industrial safety
- Modest cost, and more

Feature displays for children would show eyewear that yields (besides good looks):

- The same look as the other kids
- Durability
- Safety
- Improved performance at hobbies, athletics, and other interests
- Age suitability
- Some modest-cost items (as appropriate), and more

For teen fashions, the feature displays themselves will be more acceptable if they have their own look, and present eyewear that is the same (approximately or exactly) as that worn by their teenaged friends, but usually totally different from that worn by their parents and other adults, and equally different from those worn by those they call "little kids"—particularly their young brother or sister. For some teens, have "far-out" and "retro" styles. Beyond displaying teen eyewear that is distinctively different, show them eyewear for athletics, hobbies, protection in the sun, job safety, etc.

Feature display is obviously needed for "superior performance lenses," where there are so many choices that they can be difficult to understand. However, lens story displays in the eyewear area will occupy feature display positions (there are never enough) that are needed for eyewear. Lens displays tend to be much more effective in a separate room or area (see Chapter 8).

Perceptions and Messages

In your eyewear operation, perceptions and messages are delivered through three important vehicles of communication. You need to know the identity of those vehicles and understand the kinds of perceptions and messages they will tend to deliver most effectively. The three vehicles of communication are:

1. The communications skills of the staff
2. The look of the eyewear area
3. The feature displays

Each of these conveyors of communication will have its own or shared responsibilities in the essential task of *reinforcing positive perceptions of your eyewear area and its services*, as listed and discussed below:

- *Communication skills of the staff.* Because eyewear staff tend to be involved in the presentation of *all* perceptions and messages in the eyewear operation, there will be no list of those to be conveyed by them alone. However, the kinds of communications that will be handled best by combinations of the three above contributors and by feature displays alone are suggested in the lists that follow.
- Eyewear area perceptions to be won by all three of the above vehicles of communication are, as also listed earlier in a different context:
  "This is a promising place to get glasses."
  "This place seems different, interesting. A lot sure is happening in glasses."

"They know and care how I feel about wearing glasses. Finally, here are some people who 'get it,' that most of us don't want to be seen in glasses.

"These look pretty good. They seem to know about looking good in glasses."

"This is a friendly place."

"Most everything here feels right to me." (It's right for local demographics.)

"I'm really not interested in trying a discount place."

- Patient perceptions about eyewear and the eyewear area to be won by feature displays alone are:

    "This place is 'with-it,' right up to date. I won't do better elsewhere."

    "This place has lots of new lenses."

    "They have glasses for what I do."

    "At least the people in these pictures look good in glasses."

    "These are the Unisex frames," (etc.)

    "They've got some bargains" (items that are "on sale")

    "So this is why some of these frames cost more."

    "Look at all these 'designer' name frames."

    "These are the most popular styles these days."

    "Here's the new 'look,' and the 'in' colors. Interesting!"

    "These are the latest releases. It's nice to know what's new."

    "Should I have safety glasses for my _____?"

    "I'd kind of like to have these for when I get all dressed up."

In the above list, you may notice that there is no attempt to get a response to the question of enough frames. That's because patient interest stimulated by the feature displays should usually replace thoughts about the number of frames. (This would be a good question for a survey.) Displays that are truly interesting, intriguing, promising, compelling ("have positive impact"), can fill the patient with warm and confident feelings, including joy, hope, and anticipation of happiness, as well as curiosity and a determination to look better than ever before in glasses.

As you know, patient enthusiasm creates referrals. Patients who really like everything about your practice, including your eyewear area (where they got glasses), will want to brag about you. Their ego will often be the dominant motive for wanting to praise you because they will really be bragging about themselves for being so smart that they chose you as *their* eye doctor. Most of us like telling that kind of story. And it builds your practice.

The powerful publicity from word-of-mouth might reduce the pull of competitors offering reduced cost. Or, it could give you strength to help you in negotiations with third-party payers. If patients see evidence of your excellence in many things, including the appearance of your facility, or if some respected or admired friends tell former patients that they are missing something outstanding by not coming to you, third-party contracts might be modified in your favor, or even avoided.

Check colleague experience in areas with active third-party plans. Your colleague's project may have been undertaken to meet or at least minimize the challenge of a third-party plan. Did your colleagues have increases in patient referrals that resulted mainly from their impressive new facilities? Was their move followed by better than usual practice growth? What was the role of referrals in that growth? If that practice is thriving, you have impartial evidence that third-party plan damage can be minimized, met, or perhaps even reversed, usually with patient referrals playing a significant part.

Signature Eyewear

As you know, and has been mentioned often here, signature (branded) eyewear has unexpectedly and dramatically changed ophthalmic dispensing by generating unprecedented public interest, support, and even excitement.

Signature eyewear has already earned the right to feature display positions for presenting at least the best of your signature lines, so it will be to your advantage to have a lot of these signature eyewear feature displays, probably as many as your space permits. Your designer should be instructed to maximize the number of these displays in your eyewear area, while still allowing space for displays of other eyewear.

Each signature eyewear feature display unit (one for each brand), should contain:

- A backlighted panel carrying the signature logo
- A backlighted photo presenting that signature style (emphasizing its mystique)
- A modest number of frames (perhaps four to twelve)
- Perhaps a prop of another kind of fashion or glamour item from the same celebrity (kerchief, hat, bottle of perfume, piece of jewelry, etc.)

The eye-catching strength of backlighted signature logos gives impact to these displays and tells patients that this is unusually interesting eyewear, deserving dynamic presentation.

If you make your signature display units uniform in all important details, but different from all your other feature displays in size, shape, and appearance, you will benefit.

First, there will be immediate patient recognition of this impressive and extensive representation of branded eyewear in your practice.

Second, you will have valuable flexibility in the placement of each of your signature items, a flexibility possible because all your feature display units will be identical in size and shape of light box holder, etc., permitting your uniformly sized backlighted logos, photographs, and display items to be relocated freely among the display units as needed.

Some display positions will be stronger than others. Flexible locations for signature displays permit you to give more or less prominence to individual brands. They will make it easier to assign the best display locations to signature line introductions. Since you will have a fixed number of signature display positions, each introduction will mean that one or more lines will have to be moved, and one dropped to free up a display unit for it.

If your frame supplier doesn't have photo transparencies of signature logos and photographs, your designer should be able to help you find sources where they can be made.

To get the full benefit of patient recognition (the whole purpose of signature products), always identify each signature line with its proper, official logo. The signature name in a format other than the official, trademarked logo will be weak and could lead to a lawsuit.

Signature eyewear interests so many people that more and more competing brand names are being introduced. As a result, installing the flexibility of display positions described above will almost certainly be worth your trouble.

Because you will want to avoid having so many frames per brand that the necessarily small displays of signature frames look crowded, you will usually need an opening order of a small number of frames per brand. However, your investment in signature samples will tend to be level, controlled by the number of brands for which you have display space.

Tell your designer how many brands of signature eyewear you want to offer. Fitting enough of the above signature display units into your eyewear area without losing too much display space for other things will be a creative challenge for your designer. Unless or until demand for signature eyewear slows, try for more rather than fewer brands on display.

It is impossible to predict how long public interest in signature eyewear will remain strong. This has been debated since the phenomenon started. Some leaders allege an absence of actual value. Others point out the success of signature (branded) products throughout the fashion fields and retail marketing. Be that as it may, as long as the high level of public interest continues, as its track record suggests it could, you should probably cater to it.

Feature Display Techniques

The techniques of feature display should be almost unnoticed. The product, message, or concept must win almost all the attention. At the same time, these techniques should and can give the displays significantly increased effectiveness, partly through creating subconscious, wanted perceptions.

The techniques themselves should be able to:

- Attract and hold attention on what is displayed, while showing distinctiveness

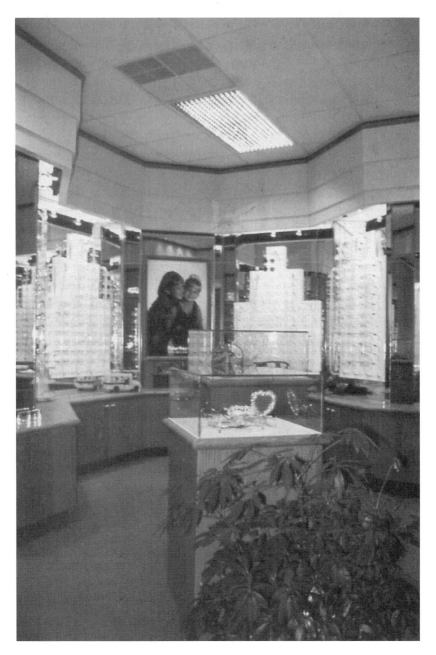

Figure 7–6   The balance between feature and mass display here responds to the range of preferred selection techniques among patients, while giving the benefit of both kinds of display. (Reprinted with permission from Dr. Chris Olson, Mount Pleasant, Iowa.)

- Win subliminal recognition as unobtrusively clever, and subtly interesting
- Support the story of the eyewear area's excellence and superiority
- Permit the strong delivery of a specific, generalized, and/or perceptual story or message

Although an eye-care practice is and for many good reasons should remain a professional health-care service, its eyewear area operation has, as you know, some close similarities to fashion retailing. Feature display techniques can be observed in retail fashion operations that share with eyewear that almost universal public sensitivity (that powerful motivator), "my feelings about my appearance."

In fashion retailing, the benefits expected and often delivered by feature displays are evidently very important. Why else would the owners give these displays so much valuable space and investment, or assign the difficult display jobs to them such as getting the attention of passersby?

Develop or choose feature display techniques that will do a superior job of: compelling attention, not merely attracting it, and strengthening patient interest in and acceptance of the information and items presented. If patients choosing eyewear can pass without even glancing at a feature display that might relate to them, that display isn't doing its job very well.

A discussion of leading eyewear feature display techniques follows.

Backlighted Photographs (Transparencies)

These proven, powerful attention-getters merit first place on this list. It's hard to pass a good one without noticing it.

Check your own experience with this relatively common type of display. Don't you almost always look, especially on your first exposure to it? If not interested, your attention moves quickly, but you will rarely fail to notice one that is well made, particularly if it is new.

For best results, the photograph must obviously present something appealingly attractive, usually bright and colorful, something likely to captivate or at least interest a lot of people. Backlighted photographs are very effective feature displays because they have maximal impact.

Appropriately used in an eyewear area, they can:

- Win favorable patient perceptions of your eyewear area
- Gain patient satisfaction and even delight with the ambience and the items
- Ease patient anxieties about their appearance in glasses
- Identify and highlight signature eyewear
- Illustrate and clarify value/benefit
- Identify specific areas in your eyewear area
- Tell your story of superior performance lenses, etc.

Transparencies as small as 12 to 15 inches wide by 15 to 20 high can be effective. Important ones could be feet wide by feet high, even in midsized eyewear areas.

The powerful impact of big transparencies adds to the area's atmosphere. Their size lets them attract and hold attention from at least the longest sight line likely to be found in an eye doctor's office (40 feet or more). Even the smaller ones are dynamic at 10 to 20 feet.

Don't underestimate the value of a few of these big displays that present the most important of your eyewear area messages so well. Even small backlighted units can have impact. And the smaller ones leave room for more of them.

By having no more than two standard sizes, as noted in the earlier discussion of "signature lines," you will be able to move transparencies and have a program of regular change. Because uniform sizes can be interchanged, it is easier and more economical for you to use transparencies to introduce new items and messages.

Because a picture or illustrated message is presented silently, the more sensitive patients will be pleased at sensing no pressure to reveal their response, an advantage for the practice. A verbal story presented by even the most experienced, skilled assistant risks having a sensitive or shy patient feel that an answer is required, leaving an incorrect perception of pressure.

Some excellent, good, and not-so-good photographs and occasionally transparencies are offered by some eyewear and lens manufacturers through their distributors, but manufacturer-supplied transparencies usually and understandably have their name on them, often in big letters. This name is essential with signature eyewear, but you may be less enthusiastic about this potentially distracting advertising of frame identity on nonsignature frames in your eyewear area.

Another drawback is that transparencies will be offered to other eye-care and/or eyewear operations in your area (colleagues, and competition). Because of their cost, choices of free transparencies may be restricted to relatively few of the manufacturer's photographs, increasing the chance that you and your competition will have the same transparencies.

There is an alternative. You can expand your choice of transparencies and have a better chance of area exclusivity by getting from the manufacturer some photographs that they are *not* making into transparencies. The manufacturer will send you a number of excellent photos from which you choose the ones you want as transparencies. You then need to find a photo processor to make your transparencies for you. They seem to cost $75 to $150 each, depending on size.

You will then have transparencies without the manufacturer's name (but with yours if you wish), plus a better opportunity for exclusivity in your market.

You might want to do this with a colleague outside your market area who has obtained light boxes identical to yours. You could share the transparencies and split the cost, so you both benefit from constantly changing, possibly exclusive (within your market) photo displays. This trouble and expense will only be attractive if you are confident that your benefits will justify it.

Mannequin Heads

Because of their potential eye-catching impact, mannequin heads can be valuable when correctly used. They seem an underappreciated display opportunity, perhaps because they take so much valuable counter or shelf space to display only one style, and because, to be effective, they must not appear crowded by too many of them, or other nearby items.

The introduction of a signature line would be enhanced when a highly noticeable style and color is presented on a mannequin head, along with a bright kerchief and/or spectacular hat by the same designer/celebrity, all identified by an official signature logo. A mannequin head will also be great at presenting your most striking or newest nonsignature eyewear and/or sunglasses, which otherwise could be "lost in the crowd" of other items.

The ease of changing styles on mannequin heads yields another fine way of promoting "newness." Some patients will remember what frame was previously shown on a mannequin head and will notice the change and appreciate your dedicated attention to newness. Change mannequin-head eyewear regularly.

Mannequin-head displays help to give your eyewear area the aura of a true fashion center, an important perceptual message. They also do particularly well at a basic function you want from feature units, winning attention to a story about a particular style.

At big shows, vendors sell mannequin heads for eyewear display. Others are available outside the eyewear field, but you would have to find a source, and then perhaps have the heads modified to accept eyewear in a natural looking and attractive way.

For maximum impact, each mannequin-head feature display should be in a place that looks "right" for it (perhaps its own wall-mounted glass shelf) and be lighted to at least twice the level of its surroundings—which means it will require its own spotlight, not too far away. If you plan to use mannequin head displays, tell your designer (if she/he hasn't suggested it) so the locations can be selected and designed.

Showcases

It should be noted that a vertically mounted (wall or fixture) showcase is usually called a "shadow box," as discussed in the section that follows. Much of what is presented in this section pertains to shadow boxes.

Originally the only eyewear displays in eye doctors' offices were showcases, if displays were used at all. If you want and can find them, they can still be useful, and age shouldn't discredit them. However, their familiarity to older patients introduces a note of caution. Assuming you plan to use them, make sure that any old ones are truly attractive and have notable historic interest, perhaps as part of your decor. Otherwise, get new ones that are eye-catching and memorable, at least recognizably more attractive than those of the past. Their success will depend on the showcase itself, and equally its location, content, lighting, and distance from eye level.

Eyewear showcase displays can fulfill the promise of feature displays, including support of the right atmosphere and perceptions. Showcases do particularly well at:

- Presenting something noteworthy (special, different) in eyewear
- Suggesting the need met by some specialized eyewear
- Delivering some other explicit message

Throughout the entire office, showcases can do well presenting an appropriate message or item (rarely eyewear when the display is outside the eyewear area) at places where patients pause and/or remain for a few minutes. This would include stations such as reception, central waiting, interior waiting, contact lens pod, lens application, and eyewear delivery. Their appeal should be strong enough to get the attention of the patient or guest there. The test will as always be the number of patients that notice a nearby display that targets them.

The usual designs of showcases are:

1. A modest sized transparent box or open surface *on a pedestal*, 30 inches high for seated patients, or at least 40 inches high for patients who are standing.
2. A service *counter* with a transparent top or full-length transparent enclosure on top, at either of the heights just mentioned.
3. A *tall unit*, imposing, with transparent shelves and strong internal lighting. These are available and are usually exhibited by their vendors at major meetings.

The smaller showcases on pedestals or in counters are usually reserved for what they do best, focusing patient attention on an idea, a particular message, or a few specific items such as a small group of frames, the colors of a new frame, a lifestyle eyewear application, the advantages of some innovations, etc.

The tall, impressive free-standing showcase compels attention and can do well presenting both eyewear and information. It has a big base for stability. Among other things, use it for groupings of related frames that you want to highlight, but avoid a crowded "mass display" look. Its high-intensity light source in the top of the unit is close to the displayed eyewear on the higher shelves, resulting in strong visual impact at the eye level of standing patients. This is highly effective but it also has a down side. High school physics taught you that light intensity diminishes as the square of the distance from the source. So lower shelf items are noticeably less well lighted and thus get less attention (also because they are well below a standing patient's line of sight).

Showcase contents, and how they are presented should be the responsibility of a creative display person, who understands the display of eyewear for fashion and function and the responses of *your* patients. That person can often work wonders displaying eyewear that is a little or a lot different, specialized, or familiar but shown in an interesting, attention-getting way.

Showcases need props to clarify, add appeal, and lend force to the story. Obtaining appropriate props will be an unending task for that talented person who creates your displays.

Props should always be at least interesting, preferably intriguing. A "lifestyle" showcase display might include some exotic rock-climbing gear, a pair of top-brand, high-tech running shoes, a luxury holder of prestige-name car keys, etc. The props should tell stories that interest your patients. For example, in a practice with a high proportion of older patients, the focus might need to be on comfort, convenience, safety, and the activities of seniors.

Avoid the all-too-common window props found in second-rate stores. These tired props are often seasonal, such as autumn leaves, or commonplace, such as mediocre Christmas decorations. Imaginative props that are recognizably clever will tend to be noticed and admired.

I once saw an eyewear display that presented frames on wooden subway track hold-down plates (about the size of a human head, with rivet holes for eyes), cleverly decked out with steel wool hair. It attracted a lot of attention and positive comment.

What about showcase security? Because showcases often contain more costly or more popular items, security can be a major concern—a valid reason for wanting lock-up showcases, tags that trip an alarm at the door, surveillance cameras, etc. You may indeed need security for some items, but unless you practice in a high-pilferage locale, showcases with obvious locks might do your practice more harm than good, by suggesting to patients that you don't trust them.

I've seen a clever, but less secure alternative to locks. It avoids the negative implication that you distrust your patients by being invisible and unrecognized as a security measure by all but the more determined/observant thieves. The one I saw was a series of showcases in a continuous glass-topped counter. Each showcase was a drawer on rollers that could only be accessed by opening the door of the cabinet below.

Feature Displays on Walls
These have the following big advantages:

- They use walls and other vertical surfaces, usually the most powerful display locations for browsing patients
- They have adjacent space for:
A backlighted photo transparency
A mirror
One or more graphics
Some props
A brief printed story, and any other feasible, helpful items

As noted earlier, there are eyewear areas where the walls have only feature displays. The try-on frames are on or in a continuous counter around the area.

Two practices, each alone in its marketing area, found that their patient number growth had flattened. The doctors decided that competition from non-eyewear services and products that were presented more attractively was keeping people away, partic-

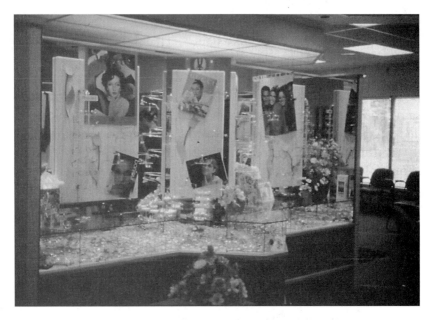

Figure 7–7   This startup, small-town practice uses feature display on the walls, with try-on eyewear in the showcase displays below. All selection is "one-on-one." (Reprinted with permission from Dr. Faye Crerar, Bobcaygeon, Ontario.)

ularly young adults and teens. Each practice moved into a new office having feature displays on most of the eyewear area wall display space. Less than half that area is devoted to the display of "try-me-on" eyewear. Both practices are now heavily booked. Their novel approach to display technique (and other factors) paid off. The kinds of feature displays used there are:

- Showcases
- Wall units
- Backlighted photo transparencies

The most common wall displays, the key element in showing eyewear in most offices, have a weakness imposed by the fixed positions of the frame holders, which make it hard to vary the display enough to interest repeat patients. Frame holders whose positions could be changed would help win attention by permitting versatility (new displays of regrouped, repositioned eyewear). Eyewear displays are much like babies. They become less appealing if they aren't changed regularly.

As it is now, any change in wall-displayed eyewear in fixed positions is usually restricted to putting other frames in those same positions, plus display aids. How much better it would be if *all* wall display items (eyewear, pictures, mirror, etc.) could be easily repositioned into entirely new arrangements. The new "look" should always be an attractive new layout. It could be focused on patient groups such as business women, outdoorsmen, teens, athletes, or seniors (within your patient group). Well applied, this versatility within displays could be powerful.

Developing the mechanics for positional versatility of eyewear and other displayed items in a wall display will be quite a challenge for your designer. Also, this kind of wall display will probably cost more than the present ones with their eyewear, props, and supporting items in fixed positions.

Alternatively, a "display wall" without positional versatility could have an attractive layout of various sized groupings of eyewear in a kind of "wall sculpture" at or near eye level. Smaller groupings could contain eyewear only and larger ones could have eyewear, and close by, a backlighted photo, a mirror, graphics, props, etc.

Feature display showcases on walls or hutches will usually be at this most advantageous eye-level position. Wall and hutch mirrors must of course be at eye level, and tall enough for a full range of people's heights. Other display components (mostly backlighted photos and props) can occupy non-eye-level positions.

On pedestal and counter showcases, the distance below eye level shouldn't rule them out, because they have proven themselves, particularly with seated patients. But for browsing patients, wall-mounted showcases at and near eye level will almost always be best. Ask yourself, would you rather bend over or stand comfortably to see something that interests you?

In many jewelry stores, window displays are now at eye level. Inside those stores, displays not in counters where people are served are also often higher, because some of their products are even smaller (harder to notice and appreciate) than eyewear. Their display design challenges are similar to those in eyewear.

The vertical span of a long wall display is sometimes referred to as "the sandwich." Above the sandwich there should usually be "negative space" (nothing distracting), perhaps with a broad line of color defining the sandwich's top. The bottom of the sandwich would be fixed by either a counter and/or a second broad line of color. Those defining lines above and below the sandwich are there to hold attention inside the sandwich area.

The other important element in holding attention at the display level is of course lighting.

Eyewear Worn by Staff and General Appearance of Staff

While related to the concepts of feature displays, this topic has no tie-in with office design. But I see it as so important to the success of an eyewear operation that I have chosen to include it.

The general and eyewear appearance of eyewear staff (in fact, all staff seen by patients) is a sometimes overlooked but valuable "feature display" that is often noticed by patients. Even with today's casual look in clothing, you and your staff should always look great, well groomed, well dressed, and with the right eyewear for your practice and its patient group. You and your staff already know how often a patient, after seeing an assistant look so good in his/her eyewear, is more confident of a pleasing result, and even wants that frame.

One successful optometrist reported that his eyewear assistants agreed to upgrade their appearance as evidence of their ability to respond to patient interest in eyewear styles and anxieties about their appearance in glasses. He arranged for each to visit the fashion consultant in a prestige dress shop, to be assisted in choosing an outfit that he would pay for within a given budget. After that, it would be their responsibility to maintain this standard out of their increasing earnings. They would also get advice on grooming, hair style, etc.

In one practice where all staff wear smart uniforms, the eyewear assistants use grooming, hair style, and tasteful accessories to achieve their individuality and "fashion" look.

Your selection assistants' eyewear is of course even more important than their clothing or grooming. Their eyewear should usually be a reasonably established popular style, a promising new one, or in special cases, a "classic," all appropriate for or providing leadership for your market. Some staff may be happy to try styles and colors beyond their usual level of taste (to be a leader, not a follower).

An eyewear assistant will often have more positive influence on patients when the assistant wears glasses because he/she has significant need for them (has probably worn them for years). This usually causes a rapport between patient and assistant. Unless an ametropic assistant (perhaps wearing plano lenses), or one who wears but doesn't have much need for a tiny Rx, is unusually skilled as a people person, that rapport is less likely. That majority of patients who are sensitive (even uncomfortable or unhappy) about their appearance in glasses will usually feel more confident, more at ease, being served by someone whom they believe "really knows how I feel." The Italians have a word for it: *simpatico*.

It can help if eyewear assistants prefer eyewear over contact lenses. A skilled *simpatico* assistant who prefers contacts will rarely if ever show that preference, but could unknowingly be less effective with patients selecting eyewear. Even in the eyewear area of a C.L. practice, assistants with no strong commitment to contacts might do better with patients, although such a person is unlikely to be employed there.

A true but extreme anecdote may illustrate the point. A doctor asked me to talk to two new eyewear assistants (their first job). One of them said, "Boy, I'm sure glad I don't have to wear glasses." The other one jumped in, "Me too. I *hate* glasses!" I suggested to the doctor that he find them jobs having no public exposure. Such foolish remarks would be extremely rare. But even if they were thought or felt, the assistant's work with patients would likely be impaired.

Do the above qualifications for eyewear area assistants approach prejudiced judgment of people? I certainly hope not. To me, it is the same as asking a one-legged person to run in a foot race against people with two legs. If you have doubts, please consult your legal adviser.

What about the cost of staff eyewear? Frame suppliers usually cooperate with valued customers, but you may be reluctant to ask often. And with different service suppliers for your eyewear and your prescription lab, you may face the expense of the lenses, unless staff eyewear is to be used to show superior performance lenses (an excellent idea where the assistant's prescription makes it appropriate). You may even have to pay for both the eyewear and lenses. As an "advertising and promotion" expense, its benefit versus cost should still make sense.

Manufacturer's Cardboard or Plastic Boxes and Easels

The manufacturer will be trying, sometimes successfully, to make their promotional displays colorful, imaginative, and eye catching. They might on occasion be useful in an eyewear area. However, where value must be established and sustained, a cardboard or similar level of plastic box or easel is a noncontender.

In an eyewear area with few highlights, where splashes of color are needed and there is no other way of introducing new styles, these cardboard boxes and easels, with their zero cost to you, could be tempting as a win–win situation for you and the manufacturer. The drawback? To paraphrase Gertrude Stein's famous saying, "A cardboard box is a cardboard box is a cardboard box." No matter how well they are done, they will still be instantly recognized as cardboard boxes, the least costly and least impressive of fixtures. Also, *you will have no control over where else they are shown.* When discount outlets offer the same eyewear as you, in the same conspicuous, low-level display units, a shopper is led to conclusions that will hurt you.

Easels made of cardboard or cheap plastic for the presentation of sunglasses and eyewear can also be eye catching and need less counter space than boxes. That could be good if they weren't so easily identified as "like those sunglass displays at the gas station."

When plastic display boxes or easels obviously have much better material and design, they can be first class, just as effective as good ones of wood or metal, etc. The problem lies with the familiar, extremely common, cheap-looking plastic units (usually vacuum formed) used to hold or display many non-eyewear products.

Eyewear display boxes need shelf space and spot lighting (with air conditioning).

Mirrors

Mirrors are important perceptual evidence revealing your standards to patients and guests.

Mirrors are *seen* by all patients. All aspects of mirroring should convincingly support your image of high standards and your commitment to pleasing and even delighting your patients.

Both the perceptions and functions of mirroring will gain from the points that follow.

Mirrors Should Be Generous in Size

Patients feel this, without thinking it. Small wall or display mirrors look like those used in drugstores in displays of sunglasses or magnifying spectacles.

Mirrors Should Be of Excellent Quality

They should be free of waves, flaws, or blemishes. Almost everybody notices when a mirror's image is *not quite as good* as in a quality mirror. Mirroring is not a good place to cut costs. Do it right.

Mirrors Should Be Plentiful

Scatter stand-up-height mirrors in the eyewear area, plus those tall enough for both at seated eyewear selection stations. A patient at a stand-up try-on display should be only a few steps from an easily found mirror. When shopping for clothing, have you even been put off when you had to ask and be shown to a nearby but unseen mirror?

Mirrors as a Fashion Statement

Mirrors are usually mounted unobtrusively, to avoid having the area look too busy, distracting patients from the eyewear. But when appropriate, mirrors can be a fashion statement, through their shape or their bold, conspicuous framing.

Mirrors of Nontinted Glass

Patients like seeing themselves looking good, so ways of enhancing their appearance in your eyewear area seem a good idea. However, it should only be done unobtrusively. A tinted mirror is usually too noticeable. Some patients might feel, "These people think my looks need help, *and* they aren't honest about frame colors." Tinted lighting can be less obtrusive, but has the same risks as a tinted mirror. Use tinted mirrors rarely, if at all, and only subtle changes in light color. (A section on lighting follows soon.)

Full-Length Mirrors

Years ago, a leading practice management consultant advised me, "Have at least one full-length mirror. It works wonders with patients choosing eyewear." Later I was told, "It's a female thing." A full-length mirror on a little-used door that opens away from the area and is kept shut by a closer will use space that might otherwise be wasted.

An Idea for Flexibility in Mirroring

Mount a mirror on a vertical post at the end of each eyewear selection station counter, so it can be turned to face a seated or standing patient.

This idea could mislead you into favoring the familiar, totally movable counter mirrors. However, unless quite large, they tend to be perceived as meager in size, which can add to the impression of a skimpy eyewear area (where counter mirrors seem to be used most often). And being so familiar, people could feel, "There's not much new around here." Finally, even though they are small, they take up valuable counter space.

Mirrors: More Ideas and Thoughts

1. In an eyewear area with men's and women's areas, the styling of selection station mirrors could emphasize the distinction.

2. The once popular magnifying (concave) mirrors for myopic patients are rarely seen today. Perhaps they are now regarded as too small. Perhaps that need is now filled in another way. (See comments on video systems later.)
3. There is a mirror that gives a nonreversed reflection. It may have novelty value, but the use of normal mirrors is absolutely familiar. A nonreversed image could be confusing.
4. You may want to use a window to an adjacent space (perhaps the lab or the eyewear manager's office) as a "see through from behind" type of mirror. Avoid it. Some patients will recognize it and resent its suggestion that you don't trust them—that you must "spy" on them.

Speaking of windows, a large nonmirrored window wall to the eyewear manager's adjacent office is a great idea, but be sure that the manager's office is so attractive that you display it proudly. If a lab is next door, a window may not be helpful. (More on that later.)

Computer Terminals at Selection Stations

Almost all eye-care practices now make some use of computers and are updating their functions and capacities. They are superb tools that strengthen practice operations, including eyewear. In a new or remodeled eyewear area, have a computer terminal at each selection station.

Colleagues can be an excellent source of objective information on the advisability of this. And computer service suppliers specialized in eye-care practices will gladly help with details.

Check with fixture makers for eyewear selection stations that accept a terminal for easy and efficient use. Or, you and your designer could develop your own station.

Display Lighting Techniques

Display lighting can and should contribute greatly to your eyewear area success. Display people tell us that more than half of display success comes from effective light levels—that it should be a minimum of two and a half times that in the surrounding area. It is easy to take for granted because excellent display lighting is usually unobtrusive, unnoticed.

Observe display lighting in fashion, accessory, and jewelry shops in better malls. You will quickly appreciate why the wise owners installed excellent display lighting.

The importance and value of lighting to gain and hold attention can be recognized in the illuminating of the outside of an entire building or the presentation of a stage play. With no lighting, displayed products become background like wallpaper. I saw an unlit sunglass display installed as an afterthought in an otherwise professionally lighted eyewear area. The key assistant told me, "Patients don't go to our new sunglass display. It's as if it wasn't there." She had the right diagnosis. Unlit displays are rare. Doctors know patients can usually go elsewhere for eyewear.

Mass displays (almost always on walls or vertical fixtures), should almost always be *spot lighted*. Don't use floodlights, as they produce an inadequate light level. To check this, experiment, by replacing display spotlight bulbs with floods or vice versa. The difference in light level will be noticeable from a distance of 40 feet or more.

Numerous "over-the-shoulder" spotlights are widely used because their lighting overlaps to almost eliminate shadows on a wall display's background. These lights can be in or on a normal-height ceiling. In a moderately higher ceiling they can be dropped to the right height by a continuous "light bar," a number of light bars, individual rods, etc. With a vaulted ceiling, display fixtures often have their own attached lighting.

There is an alternative to high-intensity display lighting. Because light intensity drops by the square of the distance from its source, lower intensity lighting that is closer can light a display just as well as high-intensity sources farther away. However, in a vertical display, don't install high-intensity lights close to eyewear at the top. The background would show vertical fade-out, dropping from bright to not-so-bright, just a short distance down the display. The eyewear even further down would appear to be poorly lighted.

Backlighting? It has one valid advantage: it guarantees a shadow-free background. However, it also creates two, and possibly three problems:

1. Backlighting makes the color of translucent plastic eyewear look lighter, so patients are uncertain about it and its suitability. At backlighted displays some patients remove a frame made of translucent plastic and then turn away. They will almost always tell you, "I wanted to be sure about the color."
2. Backlighting tends to make all colors of metal eyewear and opaque plastic styles look black by silhouetting them. Again, to understand its color the frame must be removed and held so the light falls on it. Also, metal engraving and other fine detail are hard to see against the light.
3. A bright background is glare to some patients (taboo even to promote sun wear).

On the other hand, a display designer correctly reminded me that front lighting slightly stronger than the backlighted background will eliminate the color change and silhouette problems, another accurate piece of high school physics. You must decide if a background totally free of shadows merits the expense of two sets of lights on each display, one in front, and one behind.

Feature display lighting is also critical. Use an overhead spotlight on free-standing showcase feature displays with eyewear on an open platform. Showcase eyewear inside a transparent box can also be lighted by an overhead spotlight, or by a source inside the box (like some displays in jewelry store counters). As noted earlier, lower intensity light a few inches from the eyewear can have the same impact as much stronger light, much further away.

Photographic transparencies, which are usually the most powerful of feature displays, are always mounted on the front of their own light boxes. Other kinds of graphics, and printed messages, also need spotlights.

Each mannequin head should have a dedicated spotlight, unless the heads are bunched (not recommended). Separate display props should also be spotlighted.

Display lighting is a constantly evolving, improving technology, a welcome development for every operation that presents products to the public. Professional help in display lighting will pay off, even for a top notch "do-it-yourselfer."

Display Lighting Heat

Display lighting heat, unless adequately removed by air conditioning, almost always produces unacceptable discomfort. Even halogen spotlights and other advanced units, although far cooler than incandescent units, produce this heat discomfort.

Retail store owners, and their experienced designers and contractors always anticipate and understand this, but doctors often don't know, so the air conditioning cost that must accompany a proper level of eyewear area display lighting is an unwelcome shock to them. A contractor or designer with no retail experience will usually be embarrassed. This problem and cost are unexpected, particularly if, because the project was called an office, the contractor omitted lighting from the price quote, or the designer from the cost guesstimate. You, your designer, and your contractor should know prior to designing that your practice will need "retail-type" display lighting and its associated air conditioning.

When display lighting heat causes discomfort (or worse), the doctor will, perhaps at the urging of a contractor insufficiently experienced in retail stores, complain to her/his designer, "My eyewear area is too hot because it is overlighted." Rarely is this correct. More likely the area is undercooled. You might be told, "You don't need nearly as much lighting as your designer specified. You can save a lot of money by reducing this lighting and thus the air conditioning." If that is indeed what you are told, check with your designer before you order changes.

For your eyewear area to have the display lighting it needs, and not be much too hot, appropriate air conditioning will be a legitimate, inescapable expense.

In the working drawings and schedules, your designer should supply specifications for lighting and other heat-producing elements. These will be familiar to heating/cooling engineers and contractors, who will use them to design and quote on the air conditioning installation.

A doctor I know was persuaded that the display lighting/air conditioning specified for the eyewear area was more than needed, and thus much too costly. So he cut it back, not knowing he had agreed to less costly business office ventilating and air conditioning. Even with the display lighting cut back, the eyewear area was sweaty-hot just a few minutes after the display lights were turned on. Turning them on as a patient arrived was of little help. Yet the doctor called it merely "too warm."

One of his staff said in front of him, "I disagree. It isn't 'too warm' in here. It's damn hot. I guess I'm looking for another job for saying that." The doctor stayed with the reduced level of display lighting, increased the air conditioning, and she kept her job.

It is truly important that you install the right level of display lighting. The necessary air conditioning may seem expensive, but displays that are underlighted will hurt you much more.

Lighting the Try-On Station

At try-on stations the patient's face should be attractively lighted, with no strong shadows. Patients should feel that they look good. Also, this lighting should be a little brighter than the surrounding area, so the patient feels important, which can be vital in some markets, but not in others. You may choose to have the least costly patient lighting at try-on stations, which will be the general area lighting. Unobtrusive general area lighting may reassure patients who want things to look comfortably familiar. But special lighting will often be better. If enough patients will prefer a little glamour or distinction in the look of this important place (where critical, personal decisions are made), lighting there should have more zip.

As mentioned in a preceding section, mirrors of nontinted glass and light of the right color (if it remains unnoticed) can make patients feel good, through seeing that they look good. If you prefer a warm tint, be sure it is subtle enough to be unnoticed. Why not use this tint in all the eyewear area artificial lighting so it will tend to be unnoticed and will help browsing patients?

A mirror surrounded by lights, "the star's dressing room," could be just the thing in the appropriate community and practice, or it could be seen as too much.

As always, creative thinking can yield those special touches that strengthen your practice by giving it an appealing, singular look.

General Lighting

Unusually attractive and sometimes imaginative general lighting can add to the appeal of your eyewear area. The light sources can be any desired and feasible mix of the following:

Natural Light from Windows and Skylights

Inside a building, natural light is usually perceived as imaginative and pleasing. It has a recognizable, usually welcomed quality. The fact that you went to the trouble and expense of installing skylights in your eyewear area (and elsewhere) and of leaving windows exposed (not covered to give you more room for displays) delivers a perception to patients of your sense of good taste and your dedication to making things enjoyable for them. Your willingness to give up something valuable (wall display space) in order to have windows (provided the view is pleasant, or at least interesting) tells patients of your appreciation of the gifts that nature and human creativity have given to us all.

Skylights are now reliably leakproof. Not being leakproof was the main reason for avoiding them in the past.

When there is enough space between the eyewear area roof and ceiling, the skylight will usually be at the top of a short shaft. The shaft walls can have recessed (unseen) lights that turn on when it is dark outside, or when the day is dull. The skylight effect can then continue, regardless of the outside light.

A written or verbal description cannot convey skylight attractiveness. Even a photograph is no substitute for seeing them. As you make your rounds, try to visit an office with skylights. There you will be able to see the quality of light and sense the perceptions delivered by skylights as they provide some of the illumination in the eyewear and other appropriate areas.

General Ceiling Lighting

This lighting usually comes from an appropriate number of correctly positioned fluorescent fixtures in the familiar T-bar dropped ceiling. Or, if the real ceiling is too low for a dropped one, other kinds of fluorescent fixtures would be directly on or in it.

Your designer should identify and discuss with you the choices of available fixtures, their performance, their locations, and the color of light, explaining the initial and operating cost of each option, and making recommendations. Your designer should then list, specify, and note sources for the selected lighting in the working drawings and accompanying schedules of materials.

Incandescent Lighting

This was used in the past to provide general area illumination before fluorescent fixtures became available, but it is almost never considered today because of heat and higher operating cost.

Halogen Lighting

Halogen lighting is rarely used for general area illumination. However, appropriately designed halogen lighting could highlight or give a distinct character to any part of the eyewear area. Or, it could be used for emphasis: A pool of light could be used to identify and emphasize each eyewear selection station, so patients will expect that these are service positions and be drawn to them.

In general, variations in light intensity in different parts of a single area need advice from a professional experienced in these objectives, techniques, and applications.

Changes in light level are often used to distinguish transitions from one kind of an area to another, such as less intense lighting in an access route (a kind of varied corridor), and then brighter lights announcing arrival at a new function/area, such as the eyewear area.

So, even the general lighting of your eyewear area will almost always differ a lot from what would occur in a usual business office. Here, too, a contractor with insufficient experience in store interiors, having been told, "This is an eye doctor's office," may not anticipate that your eyewear area general lighting will often cost more than standard business office lighting.

Display Fixtures

Presenting eyewear effectively and imaginatively is a big challenge to display designers.

To help you understand this, consider an exaggeration. How close would you need to be to appreciate a cobweb? You might ask for a magnifier. Beyond three or four feet, eyewear in a display cannot be appreciated. Most people want to be closer. Frames have little mass, are mostly air, and are spread out over about six inches by about one inch. They often have fine detail. Patients are rarely satisfied choosing a frame by looking at it in a display. So they examine it in their hand, and then of course try it on. Eyewear display designing is not a simple task. Now, where do you get displays?

There are three possible sources of display fixtures for your new eyewear area:

1. Reuse your present items, or buy someone else's used fixtures.
2. Buy new, current standard fixtures from a firm that supplies them, stocks them, and probably has a catalog.
3. Have them designed by your designer after consultation with you, and then fabricated by a mill-working house or, as a second choice, a cabinet maker.

Used Fixtures

Used fixtures are rarely of recent design. Although you will have the least immediate cost when you reuse your existing units or someone else's, your cost will be unacceptable if the displays damage patient perceptions of you, and as a result reduce patient loyalty. Your patients will usually notice improvements or lack of them in your new or renovated eyewear area. You will surely want patients to encounter evidence of your continuing success and progress.

If your budget dictates reusing your fixtures, consider having them refinished to look new (or better than they do now). You will need a speedy job to hold your down time to a minimum. If you buy used fixtures (either privately or from a vendor), instead of using your own, refinishing timing should be OK, but they will need to be bought well before your move.

Buying a colleague's used fixtures will usually involve the cost of your time and the trip to inspect them. And, you may or may not like bargaining with a colleague to get a price you think is fair. When buying this way, consider having the unpacked fixtures delivered by a furniture mover, to minimize chances of damage. You might also be well advised to buy insurance. Or you could rent a truck and move them yourself. A vendor will undoubtedly be fully organized with the necessary packing and reliable transportation services.

The availability of acceptable used fixtures will of course be unpredictable.

Current Model Eyewear Display Fixtures

These are likely the most popular and can be a good choice for you. One advantage of buying new fixtures from an established source is availability for inspection of the model and perhaps the actual unit. And this source has a stake in your satisfaction.

The most common display fixtures available seem to be hutches, set up for mass or feature display or both. Some of the advantages of hutches are listed below:

- They will fit into almost any space because they can be moved. Most suppliers will be happy to draw a plan suggesting the layout of their units in your space.
- Their units can usually be self-contained (eyewear, lights, storage and a mirror).
- They will almost always be less costly than similar units custom designed and built.
- The cost of installation should be less than for built-ins, but the same as for custom built.
- You can often get faster delivery.
- Being free-standing (not built-in), they can be transferred to another office if you sell them, move again, or open a satellite office.
- Under-the-counter storage in eyewear area display fixtures, which yields the well-established efficiency of storage at place of first use in the eyewear area, is a natural in vendor-

supplied units and is usually standard, but might be omitted from custom fixtures to hold down cost.

Despite the above, standardized fixtures are not always best in all circumstances.

Display Fixtures Designed to Your Specifications or Instructions

This approach opens a lot of possibilities, curtailed only by your ideas, the limits of your designer's knowledge and creativity, and your view of the larger investment. It offers the opportunity of catering more specifically to *your* patient group that should be able to win strong patient loyalty.

The advantages of custom designed display fixtures are:

- Your eyewear area can be highly distinctive, or notably different from others.
- Feature displays can be relatively exclusive, designed for the most effective presentation of items and ideas such as signature or lifestyle eyewear.
- Your eyewear area fixtures can be right for the demographics of your area, which could be up-scale, traditional, conservative, etc.
- You can have a mix of mass and feature display as varied and individualized to your practice as you believe will be best for you.
- The material, color, finishes, etc., can have the widest possible range.
- The lighting can be separate from your displays to meet the circumstances of your eyewear area, and accommodate the ideas of you and your designer.
- Fixture height can vary with high ones against walls, and lower "see-over" ones (showcases) away from the walls, for an open area with central displays.

With custom fixtures, you may reduce cost by omitting cupboards, or having only a few units with storage. However, cupboards are rarely installed later because the storage, though seen as helpful, seems to lack urgency, and the later installation adds to the cost.

Storage on open shelves under counters would cost less, but should be avoided. Even when tidy, they are inappropriate in the fashion atmosphere of your eyewear area.

Eyewear Holders and Display Backgrounds

This remains a tough challenge for display designers. There is still plenty of room for improvement, a lot of opportunities for some clever, creative people.

Perhaps some eyewear manufacturers, having invested heavily in product design, development, and marketing, would want to apply some of their design talents and resources to improving frame display techniques. It could be much to their advantage to promote much better eyewear presentation facilities (eyewear areas and dispensaries), because this is the all-important interface between their products and the public.

Years ago, when I asked two frame manufacturers about this, one prestige firm gave me the rational answer that it would be an unattractive project unless it helped their firm significantly more than others. They admitted their frustration at the often inadequate presentation of their eyewear, in which they had such a massive development and marketing investment, but were understandably reluctant to do something that would help their competitors as much as themselves.

Here are some holder design points to consider.

To ensure that patents focus easily on the eyewear, the holders and display background should be as unobtrusive as possible, so the eyewear gets the attention.

Most eyewear seen from the front is not naturally noticeable because it is almost always about 95 percent air, spread over a space about six inches long, by about one inch deep.

The specifications for frame holders are:

- Can hold almost any present or foreseeable eyewear
- Allows easy eyewear removal and replacement by patients
- Holds eyewear securely (little chance of falling off)
- Doesn't attract attention away from the eyewear

- Permits an optimum number of frames?
- Holds eyewear so the display looks tidy, not distractingly busy
- Displays eyewear in an attractive and interesting way
- Offers easiest, most convenient viewing of the eyewear
- Needs minimum daily cleaning and maintenance
- Lets eyewear temples be open

Folded temples behind a displayed frame are distracting. Patients will more easily appreciate eyewear styling when temples are open, not interfering with the styling.

Beyond the foregoing specifications for eyewear holders, there are some further needs that have, or soon will be met, while others are still ideas. Some of these are:

- Frame holders that snap onto vertical rods, permitting wide versatility in presentation.
- Security against pilferage.
- Individual eyewear facing right or left, for a more interesting display. However, patients having to step from side to side to view the eyewear could be unhappy,
- Display frames effectively above and below patient eye level. Frames above and below eye level would then do almost as well as those at eye level, the best position. The holders would position eyewear so the lower ones, at the bottom of long rods (which hold 13 frames) are tilted up at the standing patient's face, and those at the top are tilted down. This would have the added advantage that the frames in the bottom and top positions would be almost as easy to reach as those at eye level. Rods would need a concave curve in the vertical plane.
- As noted earlier, find a way of having versatility in the position of individual frame holders, so displays could be composed. This would permit ongoing changes through newly composed, entirely different groupings of related frames, mirrors, and/or graphics, creating a series of new feature displays. Placed among the mass displays, these could relieve some of their "parking lot" look.

- Glass shelves are still used and requested. They are unobtrusive. But they usually need daily cleaning (all eyewear and props removed, each shelf dusted and polished, and all items put back), the first-thing-every-morning chore of the entire eyewear area staff.
- Another unobtrusive approach has been having eyewear on either nylon monofilaments (heavy gauge fishing line) or wires (fine piano wire). No dusting is needed, and eyewear can be repositioned to eliminate gaps as frames are removed.

  Sound promising? If you have tried it, you know the down side. If the monofilament or wire is not supported every four or five frames and is inadvertently or deliberately plucked, many frames will cascade spectacularly (falling frames dislodge those below), which is certainly noticeable. Also, the supports reduce or eliminate the versatility of frame numbers per line. Without the supports, a lot of care is needed to avoid the cascade when both removing and replacing eyewear on the inadequately supported lines.

  Wire or monofilament frame displays with widely separated supports should not be used by patients. The frequent cascades will distress your staff (putting back all those frames) and embarrass your patients.

Selection Using the Internet and Video Assistance

At the time of writing, systems are available for patients to use the Internet to select eyewear from a practice. In one, a frontal face image is recorded on video in your office, so your patient can call up that image on the Web from home, and then have their picture "try on" any of thousands of frames. Once frames are selected, the patient can place the order on-line, or advise your office. On-line orders are shipped to you by the frame supplier with whom the order was placed by the Internet, and you dispense the finished glasses to the patient. The necessary installation is rented. Even if this version of Internet use proves to be a novelty, some method of using the Internet in eyewear selection seems bound to find reasonable public acceptance. You would then need space for the equipment required.

Years ago, a video technique was introduced to help patients with prescriptions so strong that they couldn't see themselves in the mirror as they tried on eyewear. A video camera recorded them. Later, wearing their old glasses they saw themselves trying on the new ones on a nearby screen.

One ingenious busy doctor hid the camera behind a "see-through" mirror, in front of which the patient tried on eyewear he/she had pre-selected, so the patient was spared the embarrassment of putting on a conspicuous show in front of the other patients. When not in use, the nearby screen was assumed to be for informational video. And because the video operation wasn't recognized, there was no problem of kids (and some adults) wanting to play with it or use it regardless of need, which would have lengthened selection time. However, the doctor took the camera home, telling me it was used too rarely in his office to justify itself. No eye doctor has asked me about this video technique or shown serious interest for a long time.

In a newer video, prerecorded eyewear is seen on the newly recorded patient's face. It is something new and perhaps efficient, as most of the eyewear doesn't need to be obtained and returned, and the patient and assistant stay mostly in one place..

Video assistance is used actively in the technical side of supplying glasses, helping to measure P.D., seg height, height of reference point on progressives, etc. Video also excels in comparing superior performance lenses to standard.

If you wish, now or later, to have one or more video units in your eyewear area, the locations and space should be planned in advance.

Signs to Identify Eyewear Groupings

Discussed earlier, this is repeated for those who want an assembled story in this logical place for it.

Your fashion image suffers when signs identify which eyewear is for women or men. Remember that your patients regularly see and buy nonophthalmic fashion items in places (stores, departments, or sections) that they see are catering distinctively and/or separately to men, women, and children.

By contrast, almost all eye-care practices have one eyewear area for those entirely different patient categories (markets) of women, men, and children. The matter is rarely if ever given any thought, but if asked, most doctors will give reasons of space and other costs.

Separate eyewear areas seem unlikely, but within the single area, different sections for the different groups are common and should be used in most single eyewear area operations. Each section of the eyewear area should present evidence supporting perceptions of your dedication to its aspect of fashion, including particularly the distinctions of gender, youth, and childhood.

Even in these days of unisex styles, the distinct areas for men, women, teens, and kids should be as obvious without signs as they are in stores offering other fashion products. "Unisex" itself might need a sign, although strong illustrations of a man and woman both wearing the same style in the same picture are worth a try.

By using decor, colors, lighting, feature displays (backlighted transparencies), etc., rather than signs to identify gender and other groupings, you draw attention to positive evidence of your sensitive response to that almost universal bogey, "dislike for wearing glasses."

There is an exception that not surprisingly helps prove the point. Signature eyewear must be identified by logo signs because that's what's of interest to the patients, the whole point of the program. Signature logos have wide recognition and are a "fashion statement" critical to your eyewear area's fashion image.

If you feel that you must use signs (beyond those needed for signature styles), make them first-class, handsome, fashionable, and well lighted. If their appearance isn't up to a high standard, they may well be perceived as a signal that you don't know and/or care much about matters of appearance.

"Budget" and "Economy" signs can do more harm than good. Most people won't want to be seen in this area, any more than at a food bank. However, the sign "On sale" is a winner, appealing to and comfortable for almost all people, regardless of affluence or lack of it.

Manager's Facility

At some time in their growth most practices have an eyewear area manager. She/he usually works in one of two places, each with strengths and drawbacks.

One is in the eyewear area, at a "control center station" with catalogs, phone, computer terminal, and other necessary items, and a desk/fitting table for eyewear selection when needed. Here, the manager is most aware of activity in the eyewear area and available to serve patients. The disadvantage is difficulty with management functions due to lack of privacy for phone calls, interviews, paperwork, etc.

The other common location for an eyewear manager, particularly in smaller practices, is a work station in the inner business office. The manager would only be there when a task required it, and when no eyewear area patient needed his/her attention. The advantages of this location are an assured station and privacy, and the disadvantage is reduced awareness of activity in the eyewear area.

In larger practices, there are valuable benefits from locating the eyewear manager in a highly attractive, noticeably fashion oriented, and only slightly business-like office, beside the eyewear area, with a window wall for seeing both in and out. Motor-driven blinds or drapes on the window wall would give privacy when needed. This inviting office would be used for:

- Work with patients your manager feels deserve this attention
- Resolving problems patients are having with eyewear selection,
- Interviews with doctors, staff, job applicants, and probably quite often, sales reps
- The business functions normal to an eyewear area manager, and much more.

A manager who is truly sensitive and talented about matters of appearance can make her/his office a showplace, presenting strong evidence in support of your eyewear function.

When the desk faces the window wall, the manager should be able to see most of the eyewear area. With that arrangement visitors will tend to have a sense of privacy, even when the window wall is open, because they will have their backs to it, and people often aren't conscious of what is behind them

It's a good place for sales reps to show their products, allowing the eyewear manager to perform this important and demanding task while keeping an eye on the eyewear room.

Because of the eyewear operation's value to practice income, an appropriately talented manager with an impressive yet functional office will be justified. It can yield outstanding and sometimes unexpected benefits.

Those with such an office say that patients and visitors who receive this "special attention" feel more important, better appreciated. One eyewear manager said it gave her a warm identity as a person patients liked, wanted to know, could have confidence in, and enjoyed talking to.

An optometrist told us that his talented and attractive eyewear manager/wife, working out of her fashionable office with the window wall, seriously improved eyewear revenue. He noticed quite a drop in income if she was away for a while. She felt that her setting made a big difference to her success, and she clearly enjoyed having this office.

The right eyewear manager in the right setting should be able to direct your eyewear area operation to the high professional standards of your practice and greatly improve your income

A Glimpse of the Future

My crystal ball is as clouded as yours, and guesswork can be a "mug's game," but, eyewear selection assisted by computer image marketing seems too predictable to be ignored. A glimpse of the future has arrived with systems for using the Internet, as described earlier. That could easily exceed the possibilities noted below.

Here is one such possibility. Each eyewear station would have a computer screen that could be viewed comfortably by both the patient and assistant. The patient and assistant would choose and call up the pictures to be seen. The computer could show pictures of attractive models wearing current styles. A "lifestyle" category in the computer could present the related eyewear being worn during an activity. As patients identified with the attractive appearance of the model (a very well known response to fashion advertising), their pleasure, confidence, and loyalty would increase. When the patient had expressed interest in a few styles, the assistant would obtain the samples, or have that done by someone else (a "runner").

If the item is unavailable, the computer would show this before the picture came up and would give a delivery prediction.

If you turn your imagination loose, you might come up with ingenious ways of showing these computer pictures that might allow an escorted, or perhaps unaccompanied browser to call up pictures on screens located at several places in the eyewear area, or in a "viewing area."

Perhaps the computer call-up could be automated. As a frame was removed from its holder, the fashion picture of that frame would appear on a nearby screen. An assistant would have to accompany the patient so the frame was always returned to the same holder.

In your efforts to improve the operation of your eyewear area, don't be afraid to dream of things that have never been done. If you are skillful (or lucky) enough to find an imaginative and venturesome designer who still has at least one foot on the ground, talk over your dreams and ideas for your eyewear area, or any other function of your reorganized practice in its new facility.

Remember that in almost any field of endeavor, those who dare to dream tend to reap the bigger rewards and often have the satisfaction of knowing they are "leading the parade."

But for now, this is enough dreaming, at least about eyewear areas.

CHAPTER 8

Design Criteria for
Lens Application Functions

Patients need and deserve to know of the benefits available to them from the recent great progress in ophthalmic lens technology. Informing patients about "lens application" in an eye-care practice fully justifies a serious investment.

Consider the whole picture:

- The superior performance lenses presently available
- The preference of some doctors to use these lenses only when they should clearly be prescribed
- Why some eye doctors may resist the claims of benefits to patient and practice
- Other elements of handling this new potential

Lens performance is making remarkable advances as new technology offers major improvements in vision, comfort, appearance, enjoyment, safety, and other aspects of lens use to the big majority of patients.

In these recent (and perhaps still early) days of superior performance lens advances, the positive responses of many patients range from "worthwhile" and "pleasing" to "critically important." When prescribed or offered, these lenses often win satisfaction and even delight because the patient gets wanted and mostly previously unavailable benefits. And the practice gains an immediate financial reward and faster growth in patient numbers.

The impressive growth in superior performance lens options comes from developments in three categories:

- *Lens materials.* Alternatives in plastic lens material (allyl resin, polycarbonate, an increased range of indices of refraction) and advances in glass lenses offer patient benefits in the following areas of performance: comfort from much lighter lenses, safety from the remarkable strength of polycarbonate material, and appearance from thinner lenses through higher index of refraction.
- *Lens designs.* Advances in ophthalmic lens design are illustrated by progressive lenses, whose benefits have resulted in fast-growing public enthusiasm. Many eye doctors now accept that progressive lenses meet their high professional standards and view continuing developments with active interest. New aspheric and atoric surface designs offer improved peripheral vision and much better appearance in lenses with higher prescriptions.
- *Lens additives.* Antireflection coating is a good example of a lens additive that frequently yields superior lens performance. Increasing numbers of people are enjoying antireflection-coated lenses because they are less noticeable and perform better. Then there are the hard surface coatings so often essential to the acceptable performance of plastic lenses. A considerable list of lens additives could be presented here, but surely the point is made.

The negative side of superior performance lenses is of course that they almost always cost the patient significantly more than standard lenses, and they often need more time for delivery to the patient. It is therefore of great interest that the benefits to patients have so widely overcome such serious deterrents.

Many doctors have some form of lens application program, as they are already aware of the benefits their patients receive and the positive patient response to superior performance lenses. In these practices, patient exposure to superior performance lenses is often largely a result of the doctor prescribing. Any further patient assistance in this area, if available, is left to an assistant who may have scant training in this kind of technical professional guidance.

Surely the point is emerging that the lens application operation in an eye-care office should be at least as specialized, well planned, and effective as the eyewear operation.

Professional Acceptance

Even when you, the doctor, are impressed with the advances in lens performance, you may prefer that only you or another doctor judge when these lenses should be prescribed or suggested to your patients—that these lenses should only be used by patients who clearly need them. This policy of course has the downside of denying benefits to patients who don't clearly have a clinical need.

Doctors sometimes judge new lens designs, materials, and additives on the not unreasonable basis of their own and patient satisfaction with present lenses. Although this should of course be considered, it could result in failure to try new things that might help, please, and/or delight patients.

Are you old enough to remember the introduction of allyl resin "optical plastic," when many eye doctors resisted it because "it scratches too easily" (a point promoted by glass lens manufacturers)? The positive aspects of optical plastic as a lens material were heavily downplayed. But as you know, glass lens use today is a modest percentage of the total.

How would the professions have responded if glass was being introduced, and plastic had always been the only lens material? Imagine a sales rep showing you lenses made of this new material called "glass" for the first time.

Sales Rep: "Glass is a fine new material, tops in scratch resistance, superbly transparent, accepts coatings for antireflection or color, and is easily edged."

You reply: "That's interesting. Does it have any drawbacks?"

Sales Rep: "Well, yes. It's somewhat heavier than optical plastic."

You: "How much heavier?"

Sales Rep: "It's almost exactly twice as heavy."

You: "That sounds bad. Very few of my patients would accept that. But I'd like to see one. Do you have a glass lens with you?"

The rep hands you the lens, but it accidentally drops and shatters on the tile floor.

You say in astonishment: "Do you really think I'd put this in front of a patient's eye? Until lenses of this new glass material are as safe and light as optical plastic, forget it."

Glass probably wouldn't have been well accepted versus optical plastic, but when we first compared plastic lenses to glass, most of us had trouble recognizing plastic's positive qualities.

Progressive lenses may be another example of this resistance. Their popularity is now growing rapidly, despite considerable initial opposition from practitioners, which was probably scientifically and experience based. If you are old enough, you may recall the reluctance of many eye doctors to prescribe flat-top bifocals instead of round segs, "kryptoks."

Your justified confidence in existing products or procedures could block objective consideration of alternatives, denying significant and/or wanted benefits to patients. The moral here is, of course, "Judge all new items carefully, and with an open mind."

How can you best inform patients in an easily understood, believable, and appropriate way about lens options that offer them benefits that are frequently wanted and important?

Lens Application Stations

When superior performance lenses are clearly a good choice for the patient, the doctor will usually prescribe them. However, when the lenses are optional, busy doctors won't have time to present the story fully enough for the patient to make an informed judgment. In a busy practice, patients for whom superior performance lenses are optional (their choice) should still learn about them.

This necessarily thorough job of informing patients and answering their questions must be done by a suitably knowledgeable and trained person, a *lens application assistant*, preferably at a properly equipped, located, and designed operation, a *lens application station*. This is a new concept for performing a new and important patient service. These stations will need everything required to show appropriate options to each patient, and to perform this specialized service efficiently and effectively. The stations must also win correct patient perceptions.

Lens application demonstration should of course only start after the patient's prescription is known, as well as their lens needs and wishes regarding vision, function, and appearance.

Where should it be done? The convenience and economy of using existing eyewear selection stations may be tempting. But this location will usually not permit the necessary time and/or be effective at presenting this valuable information to patients.

For convenience, lens application should probably be near (possibly beside) the eyewear area, but it will be done best in its own distinctive area. The "fashion" look of the eyewear area is why lens application shouldn't be done there. Lens application stations and their area should look "technical" and "clinical," like the doctor's exam room where patients expect and receive professional advice. In such a setting, this familiar process is more likely to be welcomed by most patients, and to build their confidence in the message and recommendations.

Should it be near "eyewear delivery and adjustment"? When no lens application assistant is free, having qualified technical assistants nearby could seem promising, but they would often be unavailable for lens application, even in a less active practice. The lab manager, another on-staff technically qualified person, would also be unavailable too often.

Although most of the points that follow are not applicable to design, they are included to give you a better picture of this lens application operation's feasibility for you since it is a new service in eye-care practices. These points address the question of "How should I do this?" rather than "How should I design for it?"

Lens application assistants would need to be familiar with ophthalmic optics and have updated information on current superior performance lens products. They would also need:

- Good "people skills"
- An easy familiarity with and liking for technical subjects and explaining them
- Willingness to look the part

If eyewear assistants have time for both jobs, they might be trained to do lens application, but they might lack credibility with patients when they change roles from fashion consultant to technical adviser. Also, a fashion-oriented person might not feel comfortable presenting a technical story involving optics.

Now, back to design planning. Handicapped patients who have difficulty moving from the eyewear station could be served by the lens application assistant, who in this special situation would take the necessary items to the eyewear station.

Does that idea of a roving lens application technician bringing samples to the patient at the eyewear station sound tempting for your entire lens application operation? It would save the cost of lens application stations by either making this standard procedure or as above, having eyewear assistants doing the job, working with the necessary samples, etc.

This wouldn't be good. At busy times, and increasingly as the practice grew, eyewear stations would be tied up doing lens application when patients were waiting for eyewear selection, creating serious and increasing problems of bottlenecks in eyewear selection. And as discussed above, there is the reduced credibility when a technical subject is presented in a fashion atmosphere.

In planning your lens application station operation, allow for growth in both the total number of patients receiving clinical care and then the percentage of those clinical patients who will use your eyewear area. Then, forecast the percentage of those eyewear area patients who will want or need information about superior performance lenses. Guesstimate on the high side.

The design of your lens application station deserves careful analysis. A modest and probably inadequate lens application station could be no more than a standard fitting table. However, the ineffectiveness of this minimum installation would reduce benefits to your patients and practice.

Superior performance lenses should be introduced to patients in convincing, thoroughly effective and impressive ways, perhaps as presented below.

This suggested lens application area should have on a wall or vertical unit behind the assistant, backlighted photo transparencies showing the advantages of superior performance lenses for myopes, hyperopes, astigmats, and presbyopes. They should of course also show other lens options, particularly the more photogenic. The photo could be about 12 to 18 inches square.

Other than the doctor's recommendation, backlighted photographs are probably the best way of introducing the concept of superior performance lens advantages to patients. The photos will often arouse patient curiosity. Perhaps most important, they suggest that something new, interesting, and maybe promising is happening in lenses, and the details are available here.

Further, even when computer presentation is available, patients will still want to see and handle comparison lenses with prescription powers similar to theirs, so *both* computer stories *and* an appropriate range of samples should be at each lens application station.

You might still want an identification sign (not an advertising message).

Sets of demo samples need to be extensive, to cover the steadily growing range of lens options and the prescriptions to which they apply. Your lens application station should have easy-to-use storage for all comparison samples, demo literature, and props.

The sample lenses for showing to patients with higher prescriptions for myopia, hyperopia, and astigmatism should inform them of *their* lens options. These lenses should be glazed as comparison pairs into classic styles of unisex eyewear, with one lens showing the superior performance item and the other showing the same prescription in a standard lens. Both the demonstration lenses in each frame should have a prescription in the general category of what has been prescribed for the patient. Although this may sound like too many samples, or too much cost, a compromise should be possible that will give you a workable and worthwhile presentation.

Patients will far more easily understand what they are trying to judge and be much more impressed when the high-prescription lens samples they see relate only to *their* need. It will surely confuse myopic patients, and dilute the perception of an efficient operation, if when they are being shown the samples for myopes, they are also seeing (nearby) high-prescription lenses for hyperopes or astigmats. Similarly, unless a strong prescription is involved, presbyopes should only be shown demonstration lens samples that relate to their needs and interests.

For this reason, glazed comparison samples should be grouped by prescription category, probably in handsome trays. Decide whether to store them out of sight or on display, inviting attention. Should they be within patient reach? Even when the patient can't touch or understand them, unrelated demonstration samples on display at the lens application station could confuse patients (why aren't they showing me these other lenses?).

Some high-performance lens items and standard options such as tints and sunglass density lenses can be presented effectively as uncuts. Exposed displays (a vertical, tilted, or horizontal surface) for this purpose are fairly common now, but sometimes may be used for a wider range of lens items than seems appropriate.

Uncut lens items for open display should be chosen carefully. Tint and sunglass density lenses (both uniform and graduated) will do well. CR39 and polycarbonate could be there to be picked up and checked for lightness. Antireflection coating could also be good if the sample, the background (black), and the lighting are right. A good location for a display of uncuts could be the entrance to the lens application area near the patient and assistant, or between two stations.

This display should of course have adequate lighting. Some doctors and designers favor backlighting tint and sunglass density lenses and coatings. Regardless of the kind, quality, or source of the lighting, patients often want to pick up a tinted or sunglass lens and look through it, to understand the color and its influence on their vision. Design the display for easy removal and replacement of the lenses. There should be enough room between sample uncuts for each lens to have its identifying name beside it (and a very brief story, not a sales pitch).

Lenses being shown to demonstrate their appearance should be glazed into a frame, *not* presented as uncuts which would fail to clarify what the finished glasses will look like.

Impact-resistant lens materials and scratch-resistant coatings presented as uncuts would mean little or nothing to the patient. For these cases, demonstrations on video or computer would be excellent, running continuously, or available on call-up by the assistant or the patient (people like and give better attention to demonstrations *they* control, an idea used increasingly in science museums).

Suppliers' demonstrators for ultraviolet, impact resistance, and scratch resistance should be at each lens application station. If they will be permanently on the presentation counter, have enough counter space so they won't be in the way.

Lighting should be bright, to win a positive patient attitude, and so the patient can see well. One focused, narrow-beam spotlight accurately aimed at the A-R coating sample (and with a silent on/off switch out of sight at the station) could demonstrate A-R function and benefits.

Decide whether to have an intense light (glare) to give patients objective and reliable evidence of their possible need for and the effectiveness of sunglasses, lenses that darken, and polarized sun lenses. This specialized light would also be turned on only when needed. Its location at each station would need to be planned carefully.

Lens application stations should be visible to patients passing through the "materials" areas of the practice. Almost all will notice the backlighted photos and the lens application station(s). Some would understand what is done there and look forward to their turn.

Have the most effective lens application demonstrations you, your advisers, and your suppliers can obtain or create.

Lens application stations should have a computer screen comfortably visible to the patient and assistant, for easy and effective information delivery. Equip your lens application stations to have, or at least be ready for the computer components.

Patients with higher prescriptions for myopia, hyperopia, and astigmatism could use the computer screen to view cross-section drawings of their lenses in superior performance form versus standard. Computer photographs could show the approximate physical appearance of the patient's lenses in a standard unisex frame (and/or in an edged lens shape).

I am not aware of such software or its planned development, although perhaps it will become available as the demand is recognized. One or more of the major lens manufacturers or software companies will surely respond to this need.

Such software might reduce the level of specialized knowledge needed by lens application assistants, cutting back on their need for extensive knowledge and on-going training. However, I'm convinced that technically informed lens application assistants will continue to be essential to this service, even if they are aided greatly by the welcome contribution of computer presentations.

If you are disturbed by the cost of the lens application area and fixtures, remember that this operation will be a most important new service and source of benefit for your patients, and at least as valuable to your practice as your eyewear area. That should make the needed investment more attractive to you and more acceptable to your lender.

Sourcing Containers for Demo Samples

Your sets of glazed lens comparison samples in presentation containers (for myopia, hyperopia, astigmatism, and presbyopia) should be impressive. Your standards will be on display every time these units are shown. The containers, one for each of the previously listed prescription categories (one set per station), will greatly improve your lens demonstration efficiency.

It will be tempting to ask your lens supplier to provide these sets gratis, or on a deal to promote their products, for their benefit as well as yours. This is a time-honored arrangement that most optometrists would expect and feel is fair. Your supplier probably feels that way, too.

In view of the above, it may surprise you that free samples could be contrary to your best interests. Consider your supplier's position. Although they benefit, and undoubtedly want to keep you happy, they will be looking for ways of holding down the cost of these "giveaways" (as they see them). Assuming you deal with a quality supplier, the job will probably be done reasonably well. But will it be good enough for *you*? Think of the good-looking, but not-good-enough cardboard frame display boxes that some manufacturers of good frames use to promote their valued, costly eyewear, and you'll have the picture. Remember also the story of the parachute made by the lowest bidder (a sobering thought).

By all means make a deal with your supplier. But should you offer to cover the costs? You could then more realistically expect to specify the samples and containers that meet your high standards, so they are completely suitable for display in *your* practice. Alternatively, you could get the samples on a deal, and then find a mill-working house or cabinet maker to fabricate highly presentable containers appropriate for your operation.

Does Revenue Justify Investment?

Your investment in the separate area and specialized stations must be justified by your return. Recent experience suggests this will in fact be one of your best practice investments. Revenue from superior performance lenses is rising, sometimes dramatically, in eyecare dispensing. If you keep records of income from lenses, and now actively offer superior performance lenses, you are probably seeing excellent revenue growth already. I'm told that in many practices, income from lens dispensing is expected to surpass eyewear income as a result of patient interest in superior performance lenses, not in response to orders for lenses only.

The demographics of your patient base will affect patient interest, and thus your investment, but remember that sometimes less affluent patients unpredictably choose something better for themselves or someone they love.

The evidence is compelling. One or more lens application stations will almost inevitably be needed. To have none could be as damaging as having no eyewear area.

Planning for It

Because lens application operations for eye doctors are new, there will for a while be few models for your guidance. This is a challenge to be shared with your designer and your best assistants. Explore this subject and do some preliminary planning well before you are ready to take action—such as before you need to start thinking seriously about a new facility. You have a lot at stake. Do some brainstorming.

Your lens application operation should deliver all you want for your patients and yourself, and could put you well ahead of your competition in this promising function.

CHAPTER 9

Design Criteria for Eyewear Delivery Services and Lens Production Lab

As you know, patient satisfaction and loyalty can be won or lost at the eyewear delivery, adjustment, and repair operation. The functions at this station make it vital to your success.

This is where patients meet their new glasses, their new appearance, and new visual abilities and satisfactions. It's where they bring the majority of their follow-up needs with vision, comfort, durability, etc. And it's where the rare complaint is received and responded to.

In some practices new patients' existing glasses are neutralized here, and/or payment is made and receipts issued.

Pay particular attention to the planning, staffing, and designing of your new eyewear delivery, adjustment, and repair operation. Although most eye doctors recognize that it is central to their success, it is often treated casually, perhaps because it is so familiar.

Perception, Location, and Staff

Patients and visitors should perceive your eyewear delivery operation for what it is: a pleasing and impressive *clinical* service applying the technical knowledge and skills of its dedicated and professional staff. Patients and others should sense this function's excellence and, through it, your commitment to their satisfaction.

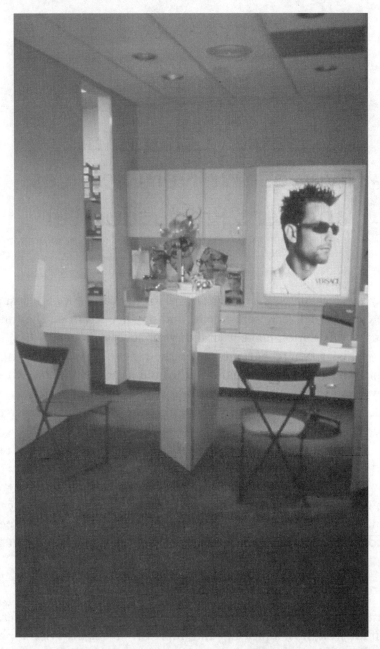

Figure 9–1   Elegant eyewear delivery, adjustment, and repair operation, with two stations, offers balance of perceptions among excellence, fashion, and technical. (Reprinted with permission from Dr. Arnold Stokol, Richardson, Texas.)

Eyewear delivery, etc., should be in its own space, located within sight of patients as they arrive in your office, and also near reception so patients needing it can be directed there quickly and easily by reception staff. An easy-to-find-and-get-to location will please patients, most of whom dislike waiting, sometimes strongly. The desire for "hassle-free" service seems to be growing constantly.

Resist the temptation to locate this station in the eyewear area to expose patients to further possibilities in eyewear (additional purchases). That would support the perception that you are a merchant, not a doctor, since the focus there is on fashion, not on clinical or technical matters. (Don't dilute the clinical image of your practice. Use other ways of stimulating patients to make return visits to your eyewear area.)

The eyewear delivery operation should be staffed by caring people with adequate technical knowledge and good people skills. These assistant/technicians will need ongoing training and updating, as with most of your patient service "tech" staff. If you don't have an organized continuing education program for them so they can have the knowledge they need to do things to the standards of your practice, surely you should start one, and be sure your office has space for it.

Capacity and Layout Guidelines

To be able to give this level of service after years of accelerated growth in your new facility, forecast the number of patients per day who will need it after at least five years.

Excellent guidance about capacity needed at eyewear delivery was generously given to me by the manager of a busy practice with a big dispensary. From computer records she compared the total number of patients who came to their delivery service for all reasons (delivery, adjustment, repair, or complaint) to the number who had ordered new eyewear and therefore came to have them fitted and delivered. The ratio was consistently two to one in a well-run operation.

For example, if you forecast an average of thirty patients per day ordering eyewear, the daily capacity needed at delivery services would be about sixty. In that situation, plan for an eventual higher number, to allow for long-term above-forecast growth, and to help with fluctuations in numbers during the day, which can be considerable. The patient number to use for planning in this example should be ninety or more. Then you will need to decide how many delivery stations you will eventually need, to accommodate that number.

Using that example, if patients average 10 minutes at "delivery services," then 10 times 90 or 900 minutes of assistant time will eventually be needed per day. An 8-hour day has 480 minutes, but allowing an hour for lunch and another hour for other things, use 360 minutes (6 hours) serving patients, per assistant, per day. Each assistant should thus be able to serve approximately 36 patients per day (360 minutes divided by 10 minutes). You would need two assistants at first (for the 60 patients up to 72, the daily limit for those assistants), and more assistants as the numbers grew.

A station is a position at a counter or fitting table, with two chairs if space permits (for the patient and a guest). Assistant and patient time will be saved if space and money permit each assistant to have two stations (or a double station) so a patient can "move up" from the adjacent waiting area to the empty station, ready to be served, while the assistant serves the present patient (same principle as the doctor having two exam rooms).

In this example, have space for four delivery stations (single or double, as above). Although only two stations would be needed at first, three should probably be there from the start to allow for early rapid growth.

Be sure you have the space to add more stations as they are needed. Your designer should show you a plan of this operation as it could be laid out for capacity.

The preceding example illustrates the forecasting and capacity part of the planning process. You will obviously have to develop, with the help of experienced staff, your own forecast of the capacity you will be asking your designer to give you.

Try to have a somewhat remote "privacy" cubicle to use for complaints.

The layout should yield operating efficiency (fewest staff steps) to reduce assistant fatigue and to reduce waiting time for patients not yet served.

Interior Waiting

Even with a highly efficient eyewear delivery, fitting, and repair operation, you will need generous interior waiting, with enough seating for patients and guests during busy periods. Also, since patients for adjustment (fitting) arrive randomly, even a well-designed eyewear delivery operation will probably become an occasional bottleneck, more frequently as the practice grows. Although you plan to reduce that problem by having expandable service capacity, a generous, convenient internal waiting area will let people have comfort (and perhaps something interesting to do) when waiting is unavoidable.

Put that waiting area as far out of earshot of the stations as feasible. Privacy at the stations can be helped a lot by using video or audio in the waiting area to mask conversations at the stations. The video and audio will also help pass the time for patients waiting, while being interesting and potentially beneficial.

Your Complaint Department and Notes on Privacy

Even the best eye doctors surely encounter a few complaints. Most doctors prefer that a dissatisfied or unhappy patient return to complain, rather than go to another doctor (except perhaps for a few chronic complainers that you wish would go elsewhere, but who rarely oblige!).

As you know, and not surprisingly, those few complaints usually occur at an eyewear delivery, adjustment, and repair station, perhaps because it completes patient care when glasses have been supplied and is the follow-up service position.

Complaints are another reason why eyewear delivery, etc., should not be in the eyewear area, which is emphatically not a suitable place for them. Patients there need to hear happy, positive things—never, "I'm not happy with these glasses!"

Even in an area for eyewear delivery, adjustment, and repair alone, you will want a patient problem or complaint discussed as privately as possible. Upon learning that this is a complaint, your assistant should invite the patient to a private place, such as (when necessary and available) the practice manager's office. If there is no private place close by, invite the patient to the most remote station, which, as possible, should be a cubicle designed for privacy. This move would tell patients the importance you attach to them and their complaint.

Years ago, one doctor used his ingenuity to get a little privacy at eyewear delivery in his startup office. It was so tiny that eyewear delivery, which he did personally, had to be done beside the entrance to the waiting room. The rare complaints loomed as a nightmare until he installed a loudspeaker in the ceiling, directly above his eyewear delivery table. He favored military band music. The volume control was out of sight under his side of the fitting table, so he wouldn't be noticed turning up the sound. He said that occasionally the scene became hilarious as loud marching music flooded the waiting room. He called it his "sound barrier."

The same idea, applied more modestly, could be useful in your eyewear delivery area (no rousing marching music or pipe bands, please). With the loudspeaker directly above the remote complaint cubicle, determined eavesdroppers trying to overhear will find it difficult if not impossible to do so when the music comes from the same place as the conversation. In any case, patients in a waiting area should be given something better to do—something more useful and ideally more interesting than eavesdropping.

Privacy between the stations will be helped, but won't always occur, simply because patients have a high level of concentration when dealing with something they deem important. Many patients receiving active attention are unlikely to overhear adjacent talk because they are focused in this way. Once, an assistant who was talking with me in a cubicle while a patient was served in the next asked me if I had heard their quite audible conversation. I hadn't heard a word.

In addition to being farthest from the eyewear delivery waiting area, a "privacy cubicle" should have the best sound absorbing surfaces (carpeting, acoustic ceiling tiles, etc.).

Ready-for-Delivery Controls

Even if you have one-hour service or some other short time, some eyewear won't even be ready on the same day. In that event or in the absence of high-speed lab service, the delivery of glasses will require a return visit by the patient.

Unless speed is critical, your patient's strongest interest will be that you deliver when promised or advise in advance that delivery will be late and a new time specified. Frequent phone calls from patients asking, "Are my glasses ready?" suggest ineffective patient communications.

Tell your designer which member of your staff will perform the ready-for-delivery functions, how, and where. Normally, a record of each job would be in your computer or on a paper system, showing:

- Its promised delivery
- Its present position in your lab or whether it is back from an outside lab
- Whether it is ready for delivery

All the work stations of lab staff involved with job tracking (including making and following up on delivery promises) would benefit from a computer terminal. The computer software would provide a regular printout of jobs that won't be ready on time, so a new time can be set and the patient can be contacted as far in advance of their scheduled visit as possible.

Alternative Techniques of Eyewear Delivery and Adjustment

Fitting tables or counters are so widely used for eyewear delivery that accepted alternatives seem rare. This traditional way has apparently not been seriously challenged for many years.

I have seen four alternatives. Number four was the only one of its kind I encountered. You may want to consider one. I neither recommend nor criticize them.

1. The doctors do their own delivery and adjustment, although assistants/technicians could also do it. The patient is on a posture chair facing out of a small cubicle, while the doctor or A/T stands alongside. A nearby shelf contains tools, a heater, etc. A wash-up station with running water is close by (to serve all the

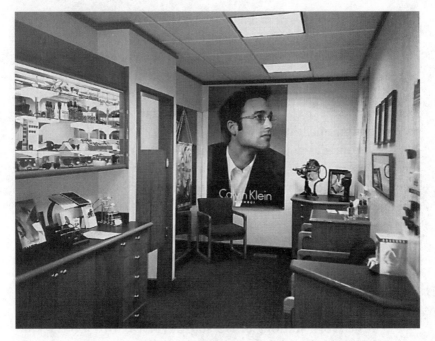

Figure 9–2 Eyewear delivery, adjustment, and repair station with no counter. Patient is seated and assistant on foot. Offers strong clinical perception. (Not the one described in the text.) (Reprinted with permission from Dr. Craig Semler, Hampton, Iowa.)

cubicles). There is enough space for the doctor or A/T to walk around the patient, to observe and work on the fit. An acuity chart is mounted on the wall opposite each cubicle entrance. The cubicles provide visual but not auditory privacy.

Patients for delivery are given an appointment and rarely face serious delay. The doctors allow time for this between clinical appointments. They value the final clinical contact with the patient, as it permits them to comment, reassure, and instruct, and when necessary, identify any possible problem that may need further attention. The atmosphere is clinical. It seems efficient, and is reasonably quick without giving the patient a sense of being rushed.

One serious drawback is the waiting time for patients who drop in for an adjustment or repair. Another may be the possible difficulty of checking the vertical position of lens reference points, because the patient's head is considerably lower than that of the doctor or A/T.

2. In a very busy practice, eyewear delivery and adjustment was done with both the patient and assistant *standing*, facing each other across a counter. There seemed to be no staff complaints of fatigue. For patients who had difficulty standing, there was one "seated" station. This technique seemed to be efficient, with little tendency for patients to linger.

The assistants had a serious complaint and a minor one, both of which were agreed to by the doctors. The bigger complaint was frequent height differences between the patient and assistant that made it difficult to get accurate vertical lens measurements. The smaller complaint was the total lack of privacy, with the patients standing beside each other. Another problem, unnoticed at first, was a patient perception of being rushed. These doctors returned to a seated operation.

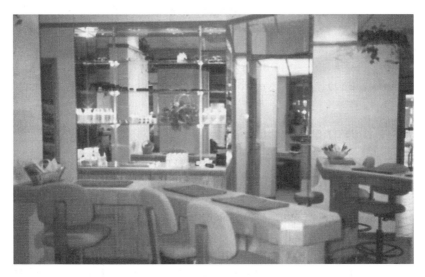

Figure 9–3   Technical and fashionable-looking eyewear delivery, adjustment, and repair operation where patients are on a bar-height chair and the assistant stands. This matches the style of the doctor. (Reprinted with permission from Dr. Richard Noyes, Marion Iowa.)

3. An unusually successful doctor whose personal style is informal (but impressive) has bar stools on the patient side of a counter, with standing assistants opposite. Patients have the comfort and the relaxed, cared-for feeling that usually comes from being seated, although some merely support themselves on the stools. Here, too, one station has conventional seating, for patients who need it or prefer it to a barstool.

Difference in eye level height between a patient on a barstool and a standing assistant wasn't identified as a problem. The doctors and staff are confident that the lens vertical reference points can be checked accurately.

This technique must suit this practice, as the doctor's success has resulted in a serious shortage of office space, a problem (opportunity?) that must soon be addressed. The informality seems more appropriate in these times when, for example, informal dress codes are so widely accepted.

4. One unusual (possibly unique) technique had a long counter at which patients sat on stools opposite a standing A/T's walkway two steps lower than the floor of the room. The walkway was clearly for A/Ts only and was against an outside windowed wall. This brought the A/T's head closer to the height of the patient's, so vertical lens reference points could be checked easily. The idea seemed valid, but at least one A/T disliked it because he was uncomfortable appearing to be unusually short.

The Adjustment Function

This operation is so familiar to us all that its design criteria have become standard. However, one or more of your A/Ts (particularly those with considerable experience) may have some ideas and want to work with your designer to suggest possible changes from the "old ways." You and your designer should welcome this. This is a worthwhile opportunity for your eyewear delivery and adjustment staff to use their experience and brainpower to improve a practice function.

One subject related to adjustments that might benefit from such a joint review is finding the time and developing ways to respond to a patient's unmet needs. Good eyewear delivery A/Ts are usually well qualified to provide this service, which helps the patient and indicates to him/her and a possible guest that yours is a superior practice. However, the time it adds to adjustment needs to be minimized.

An unmet patient need can be:

- *Clinical.* A vision or health situation such as protection from UV.
- *Functional.* Related to lens use such as familiar tasks that can no longer be done or that now present difficulties.
- *Cosmetic.* Related to facial appearance such as reducing the conspicuous look of lenses (AR coating), etc.
- *Financial.* Such as the cost of replacement lenses needed because the others were too easily scratched or broken.

Although A/Ts trained in alert recognition of and response to patient needs will be well able to perform this valuable service (another reason for an A/T training program and the space for it in your office), communications aids such as displays and sample sets are needed to improve efficiency.

The Repair Function

Requests for repairs are less frequent now. Is this a result of sturdier eyewear, or more numerous fashion-related eyewear changes? Many frame repairs can't be done because parts aren't available. However, the practice's repair operation can still be active, particularly when only a lens must be replaced or when a new frame part is available or isn't needed.

Does repair frequency justify having a separate repair position in your practice? If needed, it should likely be at the entrance to the eyewear delivery and adjustment area near the main entrance for the most convenient repair drop-off or pickup. A drive-by repair window could probably impress people, but when a repair is needed, particularly a lens replacement, the patient's record should be checked, and as necessary she/he encouraged to have a new exam, which might be difficult at a drive-by window.

In the present eyewear selection process, some patients may want to be guided to more durable eyewear, or at least find out about possible future difficulty getting a repair.

Eyewear assistant/technician discussions with patients about possible problems getting replacement parts may seem an unproductive use of time and will rarely be enjoyed by the A/T. However, A/Ts will probably want patients informed about this in a concerned and sympathetic way, rather than gamble that the patient won't be able to get a replacement part and then feel, "Why didn't you tell me about this when I chose these?" As below, there should be another way of presenting this during or, better still, before eyewear selection.

The story of how the shorter lifespans of frame design resulting from more frequent, attractive style changes have reduced the availability of repair parts could be presented by video at regular intervals in the eyewear area (or all inner waiting areas). This should reduce or eliminate using your A/T's valuable time for this.

Present that story so it is correctly perceived by patients as honest disclosure, part of a doctor's responsibility to inform patients of unwelcome things that may happen to them (as with possible side effects of medications).

Video at Inner Waiting

You already know that video is an unusually strong communications medium. Used well, it can do a lot for your patients and your practice. Used poorly, it could seriously damage your practice and your profession, through failing to serve your patients' best interests.

In the waiting area at eyewear delivery, video could serve the patient and practice in the following ways:

1. It could demonstrate correct ways of handling and caring for eyewear, to yield the best vision, and the long-term comfort patients want from the fit of the glasses established in your practice when the eyewear was delivered. This education offers the patient the benefit of fewer unwelcome return trips to your office ("unwelcome" because they are needed only to get things back to

the way they were before something went wrong—there is no positive gain).

2. It can present the frame repair story and explain that more durable but sometimes less current styles of frames are available. It could point out that you offer eyewear (frames) chosen as much as possible to be reasonably durable. With proper care, and the luck to be accident free, they will be fine long after the patient would probably be thinking about wanting something new. The patient should sense that this story, presented by video or by an A/T, discharges a practice responsibility in a concerned, sympathetic way. The video story should be so good that even a patient bringing in a repair senses, on hearing it, that you really care in all you do for them.

3. Videos in both the eyewear area and the eyewear delivery waiting area should emphasize safety. This discharges a moral and legal responsibility of the practice to the patient. One good example is the common-sense advice to avoid places where there is a discernible threat to eyes and/or eyewear, such as an atmosphere containing a noticeable amount of grit (the kind of place where the patient would probably notice that workers are wearing safety goggles). There a particle could get onto the patient's eye, causing discomfort or damage, or could get onto the lens, where casual cleaning (wiping it while dry) could produce scratches.

This video should also encourage patients to discuss with the doctor any known or anticipated exposure to conditions that present hazards to eyes, lenses, and eyewear, so safety eyewear can be considered and prescribed. An example of this situation is a wood or metal working shop, at home or in an industrial site.

4. Waiting time passes faster and is noticed less when there is something interesting to watch. Video tends to attract and hold attention. It's so strong that some patients might want to stay to see more, even when it's their turn for service. However, poorly made and/or inappropriate video can be an equally strong turnoff. For example, a scary story or hyped sales pitch won't do much for patient pleasure or be consistent with a doctor's office.

5. Interesting videos give privacy to patients and staff at delivery positions, because the video usually holds the attention of those waiting, and because its audio is usually strong enough to be a barrier of sound that masks nearby conversations.

6. A video at eyewear delivery (and in the eyewear area) can be used for "doctor-level" product presentations. You may want, and suppliers and/or advisers may urge, that this be product promotion (a form of advertising), whose common use in retail operations must be effective or it wouldn't get the space or the investment. But will obvious promotion of products, by video or other means, be good for *you?*

From my perspective, although there are possible benefits from product promotion, there is greater danger in presenting recognizably hard-sell, commercial-type sales pitches. The potential benefits are self-evident. The danger is that familiar one from the powerful world of perceptions—confusing your status as a doctor by sponsoring blatantly commercial promotions (as seen constantly on television and frequently "zapped off" by viewers).

The Adjustment Lab

This eyewear delivery operation should be organized to minimize lab use. For efficiency most eyewear adjustments should be done at the adjustment station. Most can be done as the patient watches. A few of those done on the spot should not be visible to the patient (perhaps with the A/T's hands out of sight behind a showcase display that has an opaque back wall) because the observing patient could feel that the frame was damaged despite the obvious skill and care used by the A/T.

Only more difficult work would need longer working time in the nearby adjustment lab. Out of sight there, the A/T could work without concern over the possibility of this negative patient response. Minor repairs would also be done here, but most repairs would be handled in the production lab or an outside lab.

The adjustment lab and particularly its entrance should be as close as possible to the eyewear delivery adjustment stations, for the fewest A/T steps and the shortest time away from the patient.

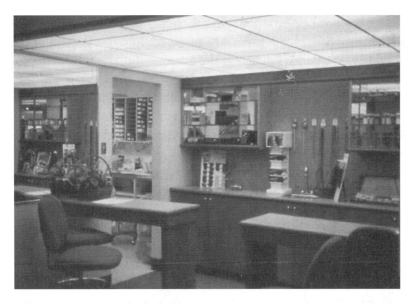

Figure 9–4 Handsome, technical looking eyewear delivery, adjustment, and repair position, with the adjustment lab conveniently beside the assistants' work position. (Reprinted with permission from Drs. Joseph Hoja, Paul Paoli and Associates, Peterborough, Ontario.)

Adjustment lab space can usually be minimal (just enough for the rare times when all the future staff are working there?), since staff visits would almost always be for a very short time.

This is not the production lab. But if the production lab happens to be right behind eyewear delivery, one small part of the production lab closest to the delivery operation would be fine for the adjustment lab. In fact, it could occupy a small part of any suitable adjacent space.

The adjustment lab needs no more than two short counters, one at a height suitable for one or more seated A/Ts and the other for those who are standing. Good lighting and at least one magnifier light will be essential. A wash-up sink is also a must, even though most glasses would be cleaned at the delivery and adjustment station using a technique appropriate to a dispensing counter.

The adjustment lab can be a good place for at least one eyewear delivery telephone, as some privacy could then be possible if the user speaks softly.

A door is optional, but usually tends to get in the way. In a smaller practice, where there will often be only one patient at eyewear delivery, the A/T when in the adjustment lab could remain in friendly verbal contact with the patient through the open doorway. The patient would have the comfort of uninterrupted attention instead of being left alone. The position of the adjustment lab doorway and a "staff only" sign should prevent all but the boldest of patients from entering.

A mirror window from the lab to the eyewear delivery area may be wanted for staff to have visual awareness and control, but there are the familiar dangers. Lab light levels have to be high enough for the work done there, but light levels on the patient side of the mirror must always be sufficiently above the lab levels, so patients can *never* realize they are being secretly watched.

The design and equipping of this lab should be planned by you, your staff, and your designer. Ventilation and electrical outlets should be correctly installed. Plan enough counter space for practice growth. As always with a lab, have as much storage as possible in drawers and cupboards below and above the counters (like a kitchen), and with knee space at each sit-down work position. In other words, this compact facility should be properly designed.

Sunglass and Other Product Presentation Displays

With your designer, plan displays for your eyewear delivery area to get the best return on investment. But, before you do, consider the following.

Eyewear selection displays in the eyewear delivery area could benefit patients and have positive results for the practice. But if they are at the stations and are successful (which would surely be your aim), they could slow delivery service to an extent that could frustrate waiting patients. If you are going to display products there, choose those that are feasible and appropriate for that location and operation.

Shouldn't patients interested in eyewear on display at eyewear delivery be referred to the adjacent eyewear area? The displays could direct them.

Patients are only at eyewear delivery briefly, and when at the station are usually concentrating on what is being done for them. As a result, displays of products such as sunglasses in this area would require strong eye-catching appeal to awaken patients' awareness of their want or need. Displays added as an afterthought can be too ordinary and fail to win attention, or perceptions, even in the waiting area. At a sunglass display, one or two modest sized, backlighted transparencies would get attention and present the message well, while directing people to the eyewear area.

Although these displays should be truly interesting and attractive, avoid making them too big, too dominant. The valuable clinical atmosphere of eyewear delivery could be diluted by product displays, unless these are done so well that they are noticed and admired, but don't overpower the area. The genuine theme throughout your practice, of meeting a need rather than selling a product, should be recognizable and believable as a message (subtly presented) in as many product displays as possible.

At eyewear delivery you will probably want to display the accessories that will benefit or be enjoyed by some patients. These accessories include chains, lens cleaning supplies, and high-quality or high-fashion eyewear cases.

If you have displays at the stations in eyewear delivery, you may want some to be patient accessible like those in your eyewear area, with others located behind the assistants' work area, so they can be reasonably controlled and available to staff while in full view of the seated patients.

Eyewear Cases

You may have a casual or negative view of cases. You may view them as just another unwelcome expense that should be held to a minimum. However, although they are often not needed by patients, and sometimes not wanted by those who wear their glasses all day, they can be an expected and pleasing part of a patient's experience in your practice.

The perceptions won by a recognizably superior case benefit the practice. The first opportunity occurs at the moment when the case is offered to the patient. To the patient, the case reflects how much you value them. A superior case is an unspoken compliment: "We want *you* to have something special." It can also reinforce the story of your standards. Even if it is rarely or never used, a recognizably better case will do a fine job for you at the moment when it is presented.

Patients who use their case should get pleasure every time they see or handle it. Most people like to be proud of their possessions, including distinguished-looking accessories.

Outstanding cases can be quite costly and hard to find. Because so many practitioners view them as little more than an inescapable expense, there seems to have been considerable erosion in the quality and appeal of cases presented or offered to patients. For example, top-grain leather cases for men are now rare.

If you recognize case costs as an important and justified part of your advertising and promotion budget, you may be doing yourself a favor.

Forty-five years ago, a young optometrist I knew bought a remarkable bargain in attractive open-end cases. He then learned a tough lesson from a patient who handed his case back and asked for something better. The doctor asked why. Without a word, the patient tore the case in half. For the first time, the doctor realized it was made of paper. The patient dropped the torn case into water, and then squeezed it into a ball. The great looking case, made of paper with a handsome plastic spray coated finish, was now mush.

In contrast, a potentially good idea for some men is an open-end case without a clip that performs as if it had one. It resists falling out of a pocket, even a shirt pocket. A case made of relatively rough textured buckskin or suede leather, or perhaps a really rough fabric, will tend to grip the inside of a pocket. I have tried it and it worked, even in a shirt pocket. Some men like clever new ideas.

Here is a fashion concept in cases for women's reading glasses, provided that the frame is strong enough to take some abuse. Some women drop unprotected reading glasses into their purses because they dislike having a bulky case there and consider it unfashionable. They could protect their lenses and make a casual-look fashion statement with a luxuriously soft (glove leather), unlined bag with a drawstring top. Call it "Belle Durham." It might be perceived as "that added touch."

These stories illustrate the importance of patient perceptions of you and your practice.

If you offer special cases, present them in a first-class display where patients will recognize there is a range they can choose from, including some distinctive designs.

Since cases tend to be bulky, storing them at eyewear delivery, the place of first use, will require planning. Store some there in custom-designed cupboards where shelving should be deep enough for the largest of your reasonably sized case boxes. Storage needs for cases at eyewear delivery will of course increase when you offer a larger range of cases.

Prescription Lens Production Lab: The Decision

Prescription production labs are quite popular in eye doctor practices. Your decision to install one in your new facility will depend on benefits versus investment, and any downsides. In that regard, the profitability of a production lab (finishing or surfacing) depends most on the volume of prescription jobs processed.

An optometrist friend with an outstanding and deserved practice management reputation manages a big ophthalmology practice that first had a finishing lab and now does surfacing. He gave me his view of lab viability. He said that to be modestly profitable, a finishing lab must process at least 400 jobs per month (about 18 jobs per day on a five-day week), and to get acceptable benefits, do 500 to 600 jobs per month (about 23 to 27 jobs a day). That picture is probably better now (lower targets) with the advances in computerized edgers.

He reports that an in-house surfacing lab is not profitable under 1500 to 2000 jobs per month (an average of 68 to 91 jobs per day). However, another authority says those targets are too high, and that adequate profitability comes at considerably lower job volume.

If your job count makes profitability unlikely, you may still feel that fast service is important enough often enough to justify a lab that loses money. The profitability and other benefits of in-house prescription lens labs have been widely presented in the ophthalmic press and at congresses. Little further needs to be added here about benefits.

There is a potential serious downside to having your own lab. Unless supplier deliveries of uncuts are fast, permitting you to make up patients' glasses fast, you will need a significant investment in lens inventory. To be profitable an inventory should "turn" at least four times per year (a $10,000 inventory should use $40,000 of lenses per year). Those economics will probably dictate that your lens inventory be limited to those of standard design and material.

You will thus be tempted to ask (or insist) that your staff use your stocked lenses as much as possible, not the better ones. Will this failure to explain and offer the benefits of superior performance lenses to most patients be in their best interest? Will it be in your best interest?

The benefits of performance-enhancing lens options and additives are wanted and will be chosen by some patients in most practices despite higher cost and slower delivery. These benefits usually impress and delight the patients who get them. Unless you practice in a clearly low-income area, shouldn't you let most patients choose between faster service on standard performance lenses at normal cost, or slower service on lighter, safer, thinner, less visible, etc., lenses, at higher cost?

My adviser tells me that surfacing lab lens inventories increase the need to use your inventoried lenses, further reducing the chance of patients being offered a wide range of choices among better ones.

As a doctor, you would surely insist that patients be offered such choices freely, despite any negative effect on your lab profitability. Your reputation is at risk when patients see and are told about high-performance lenses by friends or acquaintances who got their eye care and eyewear elsewhere, and who are wearing noticeably better looking, or just different (interesting) looking lenses.

In terms of income, the key point will be that concern over lab profit will disappear quickly as the income from your use of superior performance lenses eclipses lab losses.

A far less serious but significant potential downside to having a production lab will occur if you dislike the necessary senior management duties, or feel that you can't afford the time to give them the attention needed. My adviser said it well: "The management demands of a lab (finishing or surfacing) are much the same as for the opening and running of another (small) business." Although the right lab manager and other staff are vital to the day-to-day management and operation of your lab, you will face real risk if you avoid your "senior-level" share of it.

Prescription Lens Production Lab: The Design, Etc.

Because space is often short, plan lab size, location, capacity, and efficiency skillfully. Base size on numbers of staff, processes, and machines, after at least five years' accelerated growth. Have cupboards and drawers for storage, like a kitchen, and floor space big enough so the larger future staff can move freely. Plan bench length in detail, for present and future work stations and machinery, plus space for major machinery repairs and maintenance (with a wall tool rack and adjustable "magnifier light.") To reduce the feeling by staff that they are in too small a space, try to have windows. Lab sound insulation, sprinklers, air conditioning, and ventilation will usually have to exceed office standards. All needs for employee safety and comfort must be adequate (in the United States they must meet OSHA standards).

The lab will need correctly planned and designed electrical supply, plumbing, and drains, perhaps with a sediment trap in a surfacing lab (possibly required by environmental law). There should be running water at all work stations or machine positions where water is used.

Early in your planning, use qualified professional designing, with active input from you and the manager, plus current information from health and safety guidelines.

Rack job trays instead of stacking. A needed tray will almost always be inconveniently inside a stack, rarely at the top. With a rack, any tray can be placed in or removed from any position with ease and security. There should probably be three racks at appropriate places in the lab, for:

- Jobs waiting for materials or some further information
- Jobs being processed by an outside lab
- Finished jobs ready to go to eyewear delivery

Tray racks should also be used in the eyewear delivery operation. They look good enough and work so well that they could be in full sight of patients, while located to yield the most efficiency for the assistants.

As discussed earlier, I doubt the wisdom of a show window to the production lab. The theory is that patients will be impressed by the lab. At first, that seems like at least a tempting idea, as patients will often find it interesting or even fascinating, while getting the message of your dedication and investment toward giving them fast service and excellence on a complex process.

The downside is again in the area of patient perceptions. Many patients might sense a question: "What is this place all about, care for my eyes, or lens production?" That would be inappropriate and damaging in a "doctor's office."

A lab window would usually be located at either reception (just inside the main patient entrance), the main waiting area, the eyewear delivery waiting area, or the eyewear area. The risk of that damaging perception would be greatest with the window in the reception or waiting areas, and still serious in the eyewear space.

In the eyewear delivery area, the potential damage would be smallest. But it would still emphasize the technical, rather than clinical side of this function, and would draw attention away from more useful things such as videos on the care of eyewear, and the additional services and products that could help patients with needs that they may not yet be aware of.

In the eyewear area its mechanical image attacks the fashion atmosphere. Think of an upscale fashion dress shop, with a big inside window revealing workers cutting, basting, and sewing garments. Don't you think a visitor would have serious doubts about it as a "fashion" house?

Production lab show windows seem to be standard in one large, successful optical chain. Will you be better off with their look or one that takes advantage of your status as a doctor?

Production Lab Manager's Office

The lab manager should have an office not only to give deserved status, but equally to yield the privacy often needed for a number of his/her management tasks. These tasks include interviews and/or telephone conversations with staff, job applicants, suppliers, tradespeople, outside maintenance people, lens labs and frame sources (orders and deliveries), and internally with doctors, eyewear delivery, job delivery control, etc. In addition, there will be work on confidential computer records of lab cost, job production, personnel, etc.

It's true that your lab manager spends almost all his/her time in the lab. The same could be said about you, the doctor, comparing your exam room time to your private office time. But you know the good reasons that justify your office. The manager's need for an office may be even greater.

Being small, this office needs an outside window and one to the lab. They will make it seem larger. The lighting and decor should contribute to a feeling of space. It needs at least a desk, two chairs, a lock-up filing cabinet, a phone, computer terminal, storage, and a small closet.

Your lab is there because it delivers the benefits of fast service for patients, and perhaps a profit to your practice. Its success and the success of your service from outside suppliers and labs will depend heavily on the technical and administrative abilities of its manager. Most doctors want this part of their practice to give them a minimum of hassle. An office for that manager could contribute to his/her job satisfaction and loyalty. A lab manager's office could be a very good idea that earns its keep.

Second Flow Chart

A second flow-chart overview, this one covering the remaining steps in the overall project processes, is shown in Figure 9-5. It completes the flow-chart presentation of those processes that was started in the first chart at the end of Chapter 1 (except for the "Design Process" flow chart at the end of Chapter 11).

The picture presented in Figure 9-5 is complete but is only one scenario. Other different scenarios are possible.

LATER STEPS IN A PROJECT'S PLANNING AND IMPLEMENTING PROCESSES

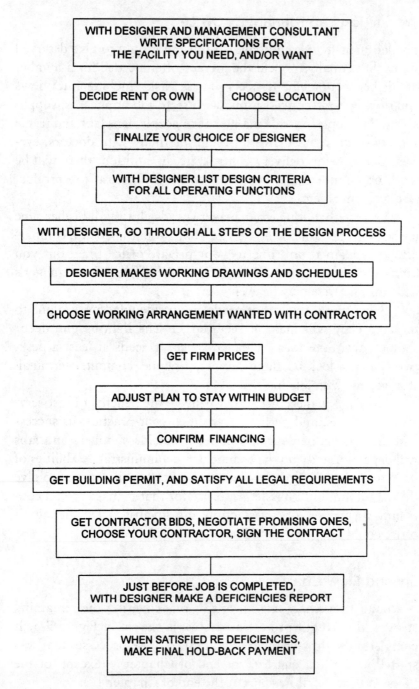

Figure 9–5   Later steps in a project's planning and implementing processes.

Nothing in this flow chart suggests the timing involved in each step or its possible impact on whether all of the steps can be included, or which ones might have to be dropped. Also, consultants in design and marketing/management are the only ones mentioned. Other professional advisers such as a contractor could also make valuable or even indispensable contributions.

CHAPTER 10

Planning an Office
for a Startup Practice

Startup Practice: Is It Right for You?

Many students and practicing optometrists and ophthalmologists give a lot of thought to starting their own practice. Some put a lot of effort into the difficult task of informing themselves. Some quickly or eventually drop the idea. Often it remains a firm resolve.

In evaluating the wisdom of making a "cold start," you will look for the best data available to help you choose whether to proceed confidently, put it on hold, or drop it. Some of your information will be statistical. Much of it could be anecdotal, some from or about colleagues who have "started cold" within the past few years. The statistical and the anecdotal may be in valid conflict with each other, and both could be right. In choosing what to do, check all your input thoroughly. You will need to feel confident about how much weight you should give to conflicting feedback or statistics.

Prior to committing yourself to this challenge, you may want to consult a career counselor who knows the aptitudes and personality attributes of those most likely to succeed in private eye-care practice. Although the advice you get is unlikely to be pivotal, it could help reinforce your decision. However, sometimes career information of this sort should be "taken with a grain of salt."

About thirty years ago, one of my sons was trying to make a career choice. He sought guidance from a professional who used a computer program to match applicants' personality profiles against those of people who declared themselves happy in their occupation. She had this data for a wide range of occupations, including physicians. This interested me, so I asked this professional, "What is the most common characteristic among doctors who said they are happy with what they do?" She reported that it is their powerful desire and need to be their own boss.

The counselor's conclusion matches my experience over the years. Although I know doctors who are happy working in harmony with others, those same doctors when in charge of a private practice have often seemed delighted to be "doing it my way." I expect you also know doctors who are individualists with firm convictions and opinions about their lives and their profession. Although that may help you decide whether you should start a private practice, bear in mind that you could be an exception. (My son was told he'd be happy as a farmer. He seems well satisfied with his career in computer application.)

Your Business Plan (Feasibility Study)

Before taking action in your resolve to open a practice, make a thorough business plan that details your goals, how you will achieve them, and all the other vital components of your venture. The written business plan will be your feasibility study, essential for project planning and in obtaining financing. Chapter 13 covers how to prepare a business plan, and the topic is inherent throughout this book.

Prior to writing your business plan, you should:

- Find and talk to highly qualified management consultants in your profession
- Tap written sources on business plans (available from bankers, consultants, etc.)
- Analyze your present financial situation, including cash flow and savings
- If you are still a student or recent graduate, talk to appropriate faculty members
- Call on selected colleagues

Getting Advice about the Decision

Don't be afraid to ask for help. Invest money (as little as possible) to get the help you need to improve your chances of making a sound decision. As just mentioned, and advised often in this book, your information sources can be colleagues, your profession's consultants in management/marketing, facility planning and office design, journals, lectures, textbooks, etc. Some sources may not be as pertinent to you as you will need, since the circumstances of each startup can be so different.

The key choices will surround answers to the question, "What will be needed to ensure my survival, and then success?" You will in fact be identifying and then expanding the areas of information needed in a feasible scenario for your startup practice (where, when, how, etc.).

You will be making the choices, so be sure you have or develop confidence in your ability to make good decisions. Despite the excellence of your advisers, eventually, the buck stops with you.

If careful analysis and reliable advice reveal a negative picture, you may decide, "This is clearly not (yet?) the time for me to start." Don't be uneasy with your carefully made decision. Even though an adviser might urge, "Go for it," you have to be comfortable with *your* decision.

When your investigation and reliable advisers indicate that your startup income should secure your survival, and you feel reasonably good about that conclusion, you should probably proceed with cautious, alert confidence.

Compromises to Accept and Reject

Even when there is no small community clearly eager for your services (or you don't want to live in one) and there is no apparent, reliable basis for your practice to grow faster than usual, you can help ensure your survival and then success by making sure that the things under your control are done right.

You will almost always be looking for cost-saving compromises. Below is a list of startup cost components that could be tempting candidates for your cost-cutting list. Each item has comments on its advisability for cost saving.

Office Location

Choosing a location to save on rent sounds promising, but in fact has limited validity. Don't accept low-rent space if the location will threaten your survival and/or success. Since rent almost always reflects the benefits the location gives the tenant, low rent usually signals an inferior location. Try hard to find, at acceptable rent, a strong location with positive elements: good looking, well maintained, easy visibility, parking that is adequate and convenient, plenty of passing traffic, etc. Then try to minimize rent in that good location (as described in the next two items).

Office Size: The Best Place to Compromise

Choose a space that is in a good to excellent location *but is really small* (won't accommodate growth beyond that at the start). Squeeze your practice into this seemingly inadequate space. Install your practice very attractively, knowing that when you succeed there, you will move to adequately sized quarters and have the financial strength to make it even more attractive.

Length of Lease

A five-year lease involves a serious total financial commitment. Try for lower rent on a two-year lease with a three-year option, even with higher rent in the last three years. Many landlords will understand your need and recognize that your request is reasonable, not an attempt to "beat them down." But they still may not agree to it.

Office Appearance

This is another place where you should avoid compromise. From the day you open, you need to be perceived as an excellent doctor of unyielding high standards. An office that is suitably attractive both outside and in can deliver positive messages about you to patients, guests, and passersby. This tends to be important regardless of the area's economic position.

Professional Equipment

Used instruments handsomely refurbished and in a well-decorated, attractive setting can often impress patients as much as new. Because patients are unfamiliar with ophthalmic equipment, the only time they will have a negative response is when units are obviously very old or shabby.

Announcement Cards

This is a very poor place to compromise. Do all you can to send out first-class announcements. Wedding-announcement-size cards are excellent because they are received so rarely. Don't send computer-produced (junk-mail type) letters. Keep cost as low as you can, but don't compromise on quality and image. One highly regarded eye-care educator insisted that announcement cards are critical to the successful marketing of a startup or relocated practice.

Try to get a mailing list at no cost from a bank manager, a political party, a local charity that you will support by being a "reporting center," etc. Be creative. Then, long before you get the cards, buy the envelopes and start hand-writing names and addresses (no printed labels). In each envelope, along with the announcement, put two of your professional cards for family members to carry easily in a wallet or purse. This will demonstrate that you are an intelligent, caring person.

Ads in a small community newspaper go in front of the right audience, but how many people will get your message? These ads can be useful for follow-up, and are economical, but don't depend on them to announce your startup, because handsome cards will get far more attention and give you a much stronger image.

Designing the Office

If you are short of money (which is probable), you will expect to do this yourself, on the assumption that the cost of hiring a designer will be completely beyond your budget. This should be checked thoroughly, because you have so much at stake (survival, adequate income, taking care of your family, etc.).

Examine your cost–benefit picture to decide how much design cost will be too much. Consider looking for a designer experienced with startup designs in your profession, who has a low fee for recent graduate startups, a fee probably based on a limited service program (for example, few or no visits, few fully designed revisions, and a response to the seriously reduced design needs of a small practice). If the cost permits your interest, check the designer's work in startup offices before deciding whether to use this one, some other, or "do it yourself." Such a designer should be able to refer you to some startup practices she/he designed, and you may know of others.

Visits to colleagues will let you check your perceptions of their designs, both the outside and inside of the practice, and get their answers about their startup. This could provide guidance (pro or con) that you could obtain no other way, giving you excellent input on ideas, options, materials and their sources, costs, and much more. If you plan to do your own designing, these visits could help you decide whether to try for an acceptable arrangement with a designer.

A designer or architect experienced with startup offices in your profession should know how to get more from a small space and how to make function spaces look larger. They should also know how to create office appearance that wins perceptions central to practice success.

Installing the Office

The "leasehold improvements" (a common phrase in designing and contracting rented space) for installing your practice are a promising but not easy area for cost-cutting compromise.

If there is ample time for a less speedy method of construction it can be done by the doctor, relatives, and friends if they really have the skills and time, sometimes at material cost (this way tends to be slower). This crew might be able to do some of the "skilled trade" jobs (wiring, plumbing, air conditioning, ventilation, etc.). All of them will have to understand clearly that this is a serious project to be done well and quickly.

Remember to check local by-laws and codes so you avoid liability problems. Also remember to obtain a building permit.

Carpeting, window treatments, plumbing, lighting fixtures, etc., can be inexpensive, which probably means they will be less durable. This is great, unless they then won't look good enough. They probably won't have to last more than a few years before your success will dictate a move, at which time better, probably more attractive, longer-lasting items can and should be afforded.

Try not to skimp on the *appearance* of most leasehold improvements and fixtures in places such as your reception area,

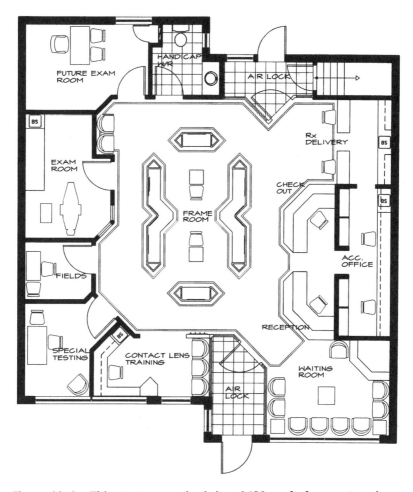

Figure 10–1   This startup practice is in a 1480 sq. ft. former store in a two-store building, adjacent to a downtown parking lot (thus front and rear patient entrances) in a town of 1800 people that formerly had a visiting O.D. (Reprinted with permission from Dr. Faye Crerar, Bobcaygeon, Ontario.)

your examination room, your equipment, and your eyewear area displays and lighting. And don't skimp on the air conditioning to remove the unavoidable heat from that essential display lighting.

Finding a Good Location

Chapter 5, "Choosing the Right Location," presents a checklist of important factors in an eye doctor's choice of location. With a startup, the priority of those factors will usually be specific to your startup needs. Those factors are:

- Visibility – high priority
- Traffic passing – high priority
- Perceptions of your practice – high priority
- Parking – high priority
- Cost – high priority
- Financing – probably high priority
- Population of the area – important but may not be high priority
- Timing in the life of your practice – this is a startup
- How much space – often deliberately too small
- How far you can move safely – this is a startup, not a move
- Whether you should be in a shopping center – cost may make it unfeasible
- Whether you should be on a main or side street – optimum visibility without sacrificing good parking
- Whether you should expand your present facility – this is a startup
- What is available to purchase or rent – always high priority

With a startup, you will usually be looking for a feasible location that will seriously help your survival and then your success in your chosen mode of practice.

Obviously, your income should climb fastest when you locate where your profession's services are in short supply and/or there is a reliable reason why enough people will come to you. For example, this could be a community or neighborhood where you and your family are well known, or where there is a strong ethnic connection.

Find a location where the landlord's interest in your ability to pay the rent is combined with a valid way of helping you. A health-care building owned by physicians has this promising potential. By referring patients to you, these doctor/owners can make all the difference to your growth during startup, thus making sure you can pay the rent.

An employed optometrist found such a building in a community near the large city where he worked. He rented two small rooms from the doctor owners. He was there one day a week (his day off from his job). The physician owners noticed that even at one day a week, he was in the coffee room a lot. As they talked there, a friendly feeling developed. They began sending patients to him.

After he won their confidence in the care he gave their patients, they asked him, "How many patients per week would you need to come here full time?" He told them, and they cheerfully assured him that his target would be exceeded from day one. He quickly achieved a strong level of success and became an owner in the doctors' new, much larger building, which had an ophthalmologist with whom he had an excellent professional relationship. He eventually became mayor of the community.

Unless you must be or strongly prefer to be in a city, consider the financial and other benefits of practicing and living in:

- A smaller established community
- A rapidly growing suburb
- A "bedroom" satellite
- A development

Provided they are big enough to support your practice, you might be meeting an unfilled need for eye care in these communities.

In ophthalmology and optometry, practices located in communities rated "too small for a successful practice" have shown consistently that a good eye doctor who is *perceived* to be good can do very well. For example a community of fewer than 700 nicely supports a two-brother optometric practice. The area from which they can reasonably expect to draw patients (their "drawing area") is much larger, of course, but it also contains other good optometrists, and within about thirty miles there is a small

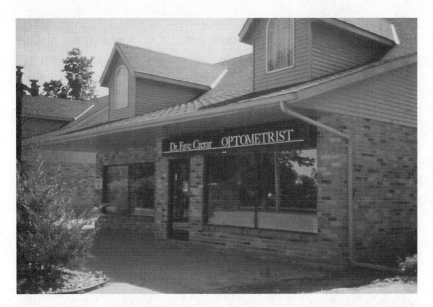

Figure 10–2 The appearance of this startup practice in a rented former store needed to be attractive and as nonretail as the budget would permit. The front window exposes the waiting room and reception, not the eyewear area. (Reprinted with permission from Dr. Faye Crerar, Bobcaygeon, Ontario.)

city with a long-established university medical faculty and a few strong practices of ophthalmology. The brothers have family in their area, but made a cold start where the population is judged "far too small to support one O.D." Clearly, their success was based on public recognition of how good they are.

In another scenario, a retired optometrist targeted communities of 1200 to 1500 people where there was no eye care, remote from a city or big town. He had sold his successful practice and wanted to cold start another, to have modest income combined with lots of time off. He found numerous possible places.

I went with him on one visit, which was revealing. The mayor and a local contractor met and greeted him cordially, and when told that my friend wanted to work a reduced day, week, and year, encouraged him to come. My friend asked if there was a suitable location. The mayor said, "You can have space in our clinic at modest rental, and we would help you find housing. We will also help you with startup costs." Clearly, the mayor and his council wanted eye-care service in their community.

To my surprise, the doctor turned it down. Later he found an even more attractive opportunity elsewhere, where he became so busy he had trouble getting the time off he desired (he didn't want an associate).

In a place where you are clearly needed and wanted, success can come fast.

Recruiting Potential Boosters

A clever way of getting a base of committed influential boosters is to use the personal contacts you make in your investigation of an area you are considering. An optometrist I know had the initiative to do this.

On almost every day off, he visited the area he favored. He called on physicians, dentists, pharmacists, bankers, business owners, real estate agents, and all others he could find time for, who owned or operated a practice or business there. He introduced himself, explained that he liked the community, wanted to open a practice there, and hoped they could spare a few minutes to advise him. Almost all gave him time and advice generously. All favored his idea of starting in the area. He also hoped that one might know of a soon-to-be-available space, not yet known to real estate agents, but that didn't happen.

After advising him to come, they wanted his success even more than usual, because that would confirm the wisdom of their advice. So they became active, sometimes ardent boosters.

This enterprising optometrist kept a list of the considerable number of people he met. Then, after he had leased his space, he called on all of them to thank them for their advice, and to give each of them a handful of professional cards.

People usually like being asked for and giving advice, and having it followed successfully. It makes them feel good about themselves. However, being asked to *help* (rather than advise) may be far less welcome.

For the giver to perceive that you have asked for "advice," you must do it before you have signed even an offer to lease. If your visit to these people is *after* you are committed to going there, or even worse, after you have opened your practice, you'll be perceived to be asking for their *help* rather than their advice. You would often be welcomed, sometimes cordially, but without the same level of commitment to support you.

You will usually benefit from visiting local optometrists and/or ophthalmologists early in this program, first if feasible. They should hear of your plans from you, not the grapevine. As you know, this courtesy offers the best prospect for future cooperation, professional respect, sometimes friendship, and perhaps now or eventually, some kind of joint operation.

There is a risk that knowledge of your intentions (from you or the grapevine) could tempt another source of eye care to move into the area ahead of you. Or, existing practices could strengthen their positions and thus reduce your chances. It will be difficult or impossible to predict what these colleagues and others will do. If one of them does this, you could still move in and succeed through the support of those who advised you to come and their resentment of the aggressive action taken against you. Or, if you hear about such a punitive move in advance, you could decide to look elsewhere.

Financing

Money for the investment can be the deciding factor when you are deeply in debt and thus have difficulty obtaining financing. Money from cash flow will control whether you can live and meet the payment schedule. Problems with money are one of the most common reasons many eye doctors wanting to make a cold start decide to postpone it. You may also be seriously uncomfortable with the financial risk in a startup.

For either or both of the above reasons, you may decide to wait until earnings get you out of debt, with some savings. Remember, though, that this is sometimes not an effective plan, because after those few years of postponement, you may have responsibilities that make you unwilling to accept the risk, and/or to live with reduced income for a year or two.

To make these critical decisions you need, as stated at the start of this chapter, a business plan that includes a reliable feasibility study for your own guidance (to find out if your venture will be viable) and to help you get financing. That study should reflect the experience of colleagues who made a cold start, and should show your forecast of income for those first few critical years, to reveal whether it is likely to cover your cost of living, your practice operating expenses, debt repayment, etc. If you will be deep in debt when you start, and you have correctly and wisely informed possible lenders of this, they will need the study to judge the wisdom of the total debt you will face.

Business plan development is presented in depth in Chapter 13.

You will almost certainly need advice on the unfamiliar task of forecasting for a startup practice. That advice may not be easily obtained. Business accountants familiar with forecasting but not with your profession may produce unreliable numbers because they based the forecast on retail business, not a professional health-care practice. Your best source may be your profession's management consultants. Get recommendations from colleagues whose results you admire, and then ask the consultant to have someone visit you the next time he/she is in your area.

Or, ask for guidance from those same colleagues. Make an evening, home phone appointment (perhaps after dinner) so they will have time, and be relaxed. Ask whether they made forecasts, and how they did it, or what their experience was with income (was it easy from the start, or dicey, etc.). Let them volunteer dollar amounts, but don't ask. But be sure you ask what, in their opinion, were the key things that made their venture successful, and what to avoid.

Even without a heavy debt load, your decision to cold start a practice will usually be made best when you have a sound feasibility study that reveals the growth in income and patient numbers needed for your survival, and whether these objectives are likely to be met.

Banks can help, but will also often fail to understand what you do. They will rarely have experience with startup eye-care practices (particularly optometric). However, they can usually give you basic, generalized advice that will probably err on the side of caution.

While studying your profession, you may, in your final years, have heard of lenders that specialize in working with new or recent graduates planning to start a practice (they make themselves known to health-care students). Before approaching them, ask about their reputation from faculty and colleagues who have experience with them. References from these lenders will be less useful, as they will tend to refer you only to clients known to be happy with them. They usually have a formula they use on each application for their decision whether to lend the money. Regardless of whether you use them, try to find out the basics of the formula they use in reaching their conclusion so you can understand their idea of reliable analysis, and perhaps adapt part or all of it for your feasibility studies.

Among your faculty or guest lecturers, there may be one or more who can guide you on the patient numbers and billing per patient you can expect, on which your forecast will be based. You probably already know who these potential advisers are. With them, as with the lenders, ask if they use a forecasting and/or analysis technique, and if so, what it is. Then ask if they can refer you to other sources of guidance in forecasting and cost estimating. One recently graduated ophthalmologist was given a clear success story from a colleague who started in a fast growing community on the edge of a big city. The recent grad found a similar situation near the same city, and has correctly based her confident decisions to proceed, mainly on the success of her colleague. This is surely a familiar story.

Before you sign on with a lender, talk to a professional consultant or an accountant and a lawyer to get essential advice about:

- The loan terms offered
- The risks you could face
- What you *can* and *should* do to protect yourself

If you reject the advice of your adviser, particularly your lawyer's, don't plow ahead. Find another adviser/ lawyer in whom you have more confidence. If you get the same advice, shouldn't you wonder if it might be right?

Take your time choosing a lender. If a lender is your last resort but looks dubious or is little known, perhaps you should postpone your project until you have more money or have found a better lender. If all lenders turn you down, you will need to choose between giving up and postponing.

Don't let the uncertainties of finding a lender discourage you. If your business plan is good and realistically predicts success, a reputable source for your financing should be out there somewhere. But in your search, protect yourself by diligence in checking their credentials, record, and reputation.

Try hard to have some of your own money (as much as possible) to invest in your project. It will not surprise you that almost all lenders will have more confidence in you when they see you are willing to risk your money as well as theirs.

In order to get financing (and for obvious other excellent reasons), you will of course be looking for ways of starting your practice that will involve the least debt. Some were discussed earlier in this chapter. Here are more.

Equipment and instrument vendors know they sell big-ticket items. To promote sales, they almost always offer extended-term installment payments essential to most startup practices. When they finance your major purchase, this reduces the amount you will need from your lender, making it easier for them to work with you.

Longer terms from a vendor would usually be more costly, but would offer you the advantage of lower monthly payments. Although there is a limit to the length of time an instrument vendor will allow for payment, you might be wise to try for the longest term.

As previously suggested, ask the vendor for acceptable looking, restored used equipment, also on extended terms. Although good enough used instruments are not always available, a thorough search among suppliers could produce success, bringing you significant savings.

If a colleague is updating equipment and will sell his/her existing equipment at a price that will still be good after refurbishing, and if you can get along without the extended payment terms available from a vendor, this might reduce your need for financing even further.

If you can't do the "leaseholds" yourself (helped by relatives and friends) a landlord may agree to help. Some do this as a matter of policy, because leasehold costs could deter a good prospective tenant such as an eye doctor. So, if you prefer or must have leaseholds done by a contractor, try to get the landlord to *finance* the job. "Finance" means that the landlord pays for the leaseholds (often requiring that it be done at minimum cost by his own contractor), and then recovers the money through an increase in rent.

Alternatively, the landlord might agree to pay for your leaseholds *without* repayment, depending on how much he/she needs a good tenant. Either way, the job is almost always done by the landlord's contractor.

There is a downside to having leaseholds done (rather than only "paid for") by the landlord. Because the landlord will want the lowest possible cost, you may not like the job, but might have to accept it because it is helping you with your financing. Eye doctors (not startup) I know have been bitterly disappointed by poor work they couldn't avoid because the contractor was working for the landlord, at lowest cost.

When financing problems are less critical, your best bet will be a landlord's *financial allowance* so you can have the contracting done to your standards and satisfaction.

See Chapter 13, the section on financing and making a business plan, which includes advice on starting, relocating or expanding a practice.

The Challenge and the Joy

Starting an eye-care practice will be a different experience for all who choose to do it. Although information from texts and other sources can be very helpful, your personal attributes, including daring and innovation, will make a big difference. A wonderful feeling of accomplishment awaits those who succeed in this career path.

CHAPTER 11

What to Expect from Your Designer–Consultant

Predesign Planning Team

For your predesign planning, two consulting services will be best. They are an ophthalmic (ophthalmology and/or optometry) designer–consultant (an "ODC") and an ophthalmic management and marketing consultant (an "OMMC"). The range of their combined specialized knowledge should cover almost all of the vital information and advice you will need.

Although my experience has been mostly in the ODC side of predesign planning, it has been easy to recognize and respect the value of a top OMMC's services.

Considering Consultants

After your first big decision—"My practice needs an improved office"—you add some of your goals: "A practice that has greater capacity, a wider range of services, is more patient-friendly, more impressive, more efficient." Your project gets bigger and more complicated steadily. Usually at this point, you recognize that you need help with those tough early planning and designing decisions, including the wisdom of the project itself.

If you choose to use an OMMC and an ODC, look for those whose services, qualifications, and years of experience in their aspects of planning expansions, relocations, and startups of eye-care practices make you confident they will fully understand and appreciate *your* practice, *your* objectives, and *your* budget limits.

The combined services of an OMMC and ODC will tend to have three components: an OMMC component, an area of information overlap, and an ODC component.

Within the design process, the role of your ophthalmic design consultant (ODC) will gradually shift from consultation to designing. When that occurs, I will refer to this person or persons as your "designer," rather than "ODC."

Your accountant, your lawyer, and key staff will already be available. An appropriately experienced contractor should also be contributing, but not necessarily at the predesign stage.

Subjects for Combined ODC and OMMC Advice

Planning decisions that affect design will be needed before designing can begin because predesign planning and designing are interwoven processes based on your objectives, needs, wants, costs, comfort with risk, availability of financing, etc.

Have both your ODC and OMMC advise you on the following subjects:

1. Project feasibility
2. Alternatives to the project, and options within it
3. Size of space needed
4. Location
5. Timing

All of these topics are presented at length elsewhere in this book and are discussed briefly in the sections that follow.

Project Feasibility

Although many steps in a feasibility study should be guided by an OMMC, your familiarity with your practice and your access to colleagues uniquely qualifies you to contribute to forecasts of patient numbers and revenue growth.

Alternatives to the Project and Options Within It

Your alternatives are, of course, your major feasible choices for achieving your objectives, fulfilling your ambitions, and/or solving your practice problems after you are sure you have correctly identified them.

Size of Space Needed

Are you considering space that is or soon will be too small? Ask colleagues who moved into new facilities whether this has been their experience or is anticipated. Although fewer than 50 percent of the eye doctors I've asked (see questionnaire report, Chapter 14) have complained, "I wish I'd taken more space," there are too many to be ignored. Get your ODC's advice on the space you are likely to need after five years. Investigate this carefully before making your choice of "small as feasible" or "big as feasible" space. Your choice will have to be personal, as each can be supported by valid reasons:

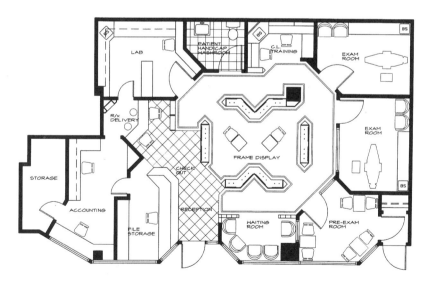

Figure 11–1   A compact design to squeeze an active practice into a small space of 1,400 sq. ft. (They outgrew it and moved to another active location.) [Reprinted with permission from Drs. Gordon Moore and David Frewin, New Westminster (beside Vancouver), British Columbia.]

- Small as feasible: because a larger space will raise project cost too far above target, because "the size and the decision about it feels right," and because you view a further expansion move as a normal, valuable opportunity in your successful career path
- Big as feasible: because you expect to outgrow your new facility too soon

Location Choice

The importance of location and the factors involved in the choice are presented in Chapter 4 as a checklist to help you "touch all the bases" in considering your location.

The choice is rarely obvious. An adviser with appropriate experience and a good understanding of your objectives and criteria should be able to:

- Recommend the best location
- Recommend the sequence among several acceptable but not outstanding locations
- Report that none seems acceptable

One busy, hurried doctor had a close call. He found and was interested in a modest rental storefront location beside an empty store. Then he found a better place. In the other location, a noisy, dirty restaurant moved into the adjacent store and inflicted problems with parking, smells, and vermin on its neighbors. Try for a locale that has good, stable, established neighbors.

Another doctor wasn't so lucky. This doctor signed the "offer to lease," and then the lease, before researching size of space among colleagues. Recognizing a bad decision (space too small) the doctor paid a modest penalty to get out of the lease (the landlord cooperated in not enforcing the lease, as was his legal right).

Try not to be hasty. That old adage has a flip side: He who hesitates is sometimes saved.

Timing

You will want to be practicing in your new space by the start of rent or purchase payments, to avoid paying for two offices at the same time.

Will this target be wise or feasible? When a deadline controls many decisions about a new office, the reduced time for planning, designing, and contracting too often imposes damaging compromises that can hurt your chances of achieving your objectives.

If you face a firm deadline to vacate, or some other tight time pressure, try to get truly *reliable* advice on:

- A prediction that the deadline won't be met so you can make alternate plans, such as a temporary office
- How to get, with the least risk, the fast timing you have been realistically told will permit you to meet the deadline

Remember, however: even the best experience-based predictions and promises of fast completion include the sometimes unspoken, dangerous qualifier "if nothing goes wrong" (which is rare and unpredictable). Even when you are advised by an appropriately experienced independent ODC, allow more time than you are told to expect.

Extensive time for planning, etc., is to your advantage, not a source of problems. But do your planning on a firm schedule (daily, or at least weekly). Without that schedule, a year or more could evaporate.

If your deadline won't be met, be creative so your project can be completed to the level of excellence needed, as in the following hard to believe, but true story.

The landlord of an optometrist I know insisted he vacate his space when the lease ended in one month's time. His present space was already leased by another optometrist. Unpredictable problems delayed the project so work on his new building hadn't started, and winter (severe in his area) was about to begin. He had, and still has, a truly successful practice.

Quite a problem! Here's what he did. His future parking lot was paved immediately and a full-sized billboard was erected at its far edge. The billboard had a full-color, eye-catching rendering of his new building, and the message, "Announcing the future office of Dr. _____ , now practicing temporarily in the trailer behind this sign." An arrow at the end of this message, on the bottom right corner of the billboard, pointed to the exposed entrance to a large trailer, the rest of which was hidden behind the bill-board. The trailer was outfitted for temporary, minimum practice. All this, although it was an added expense, cost a lot less than being out of operation.

Fortunately, the location was on a busy traffic artery.

After moving into his fine new building about a year later, the doctor experienced an unexpectedly high jump in practice income, resulting in part from that publicity. That practice jump also offset a lot of the cost. The doctor felt that he kept almost all his patients, most of whom were unusually loyal to him. Those who wanted to wait made appointments for his new building. Most chose to be taken care of in the trailer.

Why Work with a Designer Consultant (ODC)?

You will benefit in ways described later in this chapter from having a well-qualified professional ODC working with you on all stages of the often critical predesign planning and early designing, including the conceptual design process.

Choose your designer carefully, basing your choice on his/her work that you have seen, contacts with former clients (reputation), and your contacts with her/him. Have exploratory talks with one or more of the consultants, both for answers to your questions and to see if you feel comfortable with the process and the person. Once you have confidence in an ODC candidate, you will be ready to start.

The designer will probably expect to be retained for all the ODC services you will need, which makes sense because the portion of the designer's fee that covers predesign planning to the end of conceptual design can be more than 50 percent of the fee for total services.

With a small or startup project, the assistance of a well-qualified ODC and/or OMMC should be just as valuable toward your success as with a larger one, but with fees and services tailored to your need as much as possible.

Ask colleagues who used ODC and/or OMMC services whether the result justified the cost, compared to what they believe would have occurred without those services.

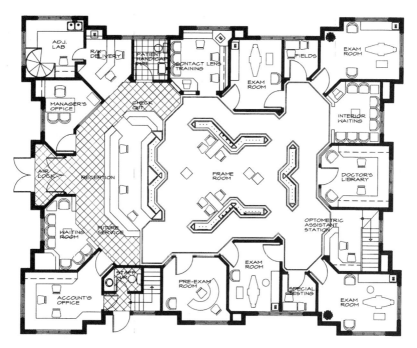

Figure 11–2 Doctor's busy practice moved into his new building in 3,100 sq. ft. office designed to meet his objectives, needs, wants, and mode of practice, including locations of some services. (Reprinted with permission from Dr. Riley Uglum, New Hampton, Iowa. Population 3,660.)

When you make this critical choice, weigh cost against benefit by finding out what is included in the process. This will also reveal what you must expect from yourself without the services of the ODC or OMMC. If you then feel that you don't need this assistance, you will have the confidence of knowing you made an informed decision.

The foregoing suggests that you not dismiss in advance (as "too costly for me") the idea of using ODC and/or OMMC services.

Another way of giving you an understanding of the more serious predesign planning and design decisions you would face alone would be a comprehensive list of the major predesign planning and design decisions in a project. However, since these are the topics presented and discussed at length in this book, much of the list already exists in the table of contents, and the story of your benefits from OMMC and ODC participation occurs throughout this chapter.

Designer (ODC) Advice on Project Choices You Make

Although responsibility for your success is shared among you, your ODC, your OMMC, and your contractor, the decisions will be yours, supported by the others' professional advice.

As mentioned before, each project for an ophthalmology and/or optometry facility is different. Many differences stem from the doctor's choices among factors that control or influence the design.

For your designer to give you the best guidance, she/he must explore and understand these "personal to you" design controlling items in your project, as listed below:

- *Scope of project.* A "project" could range from a single practice function (an eyewear area) to all steps in erecting a new building (location, site plan, and the complete design process described in what follows).
- *Practice problems that this project must solve.* Often the list is topped by, "A serious slowing of growth in both patient numbers and practice income, because the practice reached capacity," but other problems could dominate, such as demographic changes that make another location more promising, competition, time for renewal that patients will appreciate, lease renewal problems, etc.
- *Your budget limit.* This will be influenced by income forecasts and the availability of financing.
- *Your point of view as owner(s) about this kind and/or size of project.*
- *Your additional objectives beyond problem-solving.* After return on investment and better personal income, these range widely, including attracting a suitable new doctor, attracting a daughter or son into your practice, etc.
- *All your operational criteria for your desired mode of practice.*

- *The scope of work you want from your designer.* What you want in the design process, almost always based on your view of its value to you.
- *Timing you need or want.*
- *Your still-to-be-decided design specifications, and/or materials and fixture choices.*

ODC Qualifications

Experience and ability (talent) are the most important things your ODC brings to planning and designing your project. Constantly broadening experience in the design of eye doctors' facilities of all kinds and sizes, applied intelligently and creatively to your objectives, is a promising formula for a designer's contribution to most aspects of your design project.

Education is of course essential, but for you, the most valuable aspect of a designer's education comes from years of experience with design projects within your profession. In spite of that, of course, an architect or designer with minimal experience but recognizable, impressive talent could deservedly win your confidence and do a fine job.

You will have your own reasons for choosing your ODC or deciding not to have one. It is unreasonable to expect a uniform way of choosing that will suit all eye doctors, in all design projects.

Compromise in Planning

The planning and design process is often called "problem solving": creating solutions to the problems inherent to that project's particular objectives and criteria. To produce the best solutions the team members (client and designer) must each make important contributions that lead to compromises most acceptable to the client.

Compromise characterizes these final decisions. The client will often be making individualized judgments based on, "If I get this wanted item, I lose another that I like."

The Design Process and Responsibilities of the Designer up to Conceptual Design

The design process can have several major components, each with its own steps. Your design process should of course include all services that are clearly essential to your project. Components (both essential and optional) common to the entire design process are listed below, followed by details of the service steps in each of them:

- Getting reliable background information (basic criteria for conceptual design)
- The conceptual design process
- The working drawings and schedules process
- Project management

Reliable Background Information

To start the design process, your designer must obtain a wide range of reliable background information about:

- The objective(s) that control your project
- Your dream or ambition
- The problem(s) you need and/or want to solve
- The opportunity you want to use
- The practice as it functions now
- Your situation and point of view as the owner/doctor
- What has been done on the project to date

Project Information

For you to get the most benefit from this thorough information gathering, *your designer should visit you,* particularly during and after office hours. If the designer must travel a substantial distance, the best timing for this visit will usually be arrival in midafternoon and departure the next afternoon. This will allow time for the designer to do the following.

Afternoon of Arrival

Observe the practice in operation, and have brief conversations with staff.

That Evening
Have an uninterrupted discussion with you and perhaps your accountant, key staff members, and/or anyone else whose advice you value. You might want a landlord there briefly.

Afternoon and Evening Combined
Get a clear picture of the background information just listed:

- Observe your preferred mode of practice
- Listen to innovations you want to introduce
- Hear your point of view about this venture, including budget limit
- Obtain your design criteria, through an often time-consuming, detailed, and thorough discussion of the operating functions you want or are considering
- Discuss the scope of responsibility possible from your project designer, so you can later choose what you want her/his participation to be
- Discuss fees for the different components of design service that you might want

Late Evening
The designer, working alone, will:

- List options to be suggested to you the next day
- Identify possible problems (with detailed supporting evidence)
- Prepare other topics for discussion

The Following Morning
Meet to discuss:

- Suggested options
- Any newly identified, possible problems
- Aspects of the project cost
- Timing
- Feasibility if it seems uncertain

and other topics. The face-to-face meetings central to a visit will enable the best interaction between you. These meetings will be vital to the critical task of identifying and understanding your design criteria (the detailed list of the functions you want, and the specifics of how they will operate in your new or renovated facility). The design criteria form the essential base for the designer's first conceptual design, presented in a section that follows, "The Conceptual Design Process."

The cost of this visit is usually seen as fine value in terms of your benefits from those first conceptual design process steps (e.g., analysis of design criteria in face-to-face meetings when communication is usually at its best, and the information gathering done by the designer from observation and conversation with your assistants).

There is another, frequently used, much less costly method of getting information. The design firm sends a comprehensive questionnaire for you to answer. After they review your answers, either the designer or another key person at the design source discusses them and the other pertinent topics with you in one or more phone calls. Although the results obtained this way will rarely be as thorough as those obtained from a visit, the widespread use of this method indicates its popularity—probably because of the cost savings, and because clients find that it does an acceptable job. Once again, we suggest that you check this with colleagues.

Problems to Be Solved and Your "Other Objectives"

As discussed earlier, the ODC and the OMMC should get the story and details of any practice problems that initiated this project. Working with you, they should examine and evaluate these problems, advise on the feasibility of proposed solutions, and suggest workable alternatives—even, on rare occasions, the alternative of abandoning or postponing the project.

Your Situation and Views as Doctor/Owner

This includes those circumstances you face and your firmly held views that could enhance or threaten project success or feasibility. These are in part:

- Obligations to, and relationships with a partner
- Present financial position (debt, borrowing power, etc.)

- The timing of any retirement plans you may have in mind
- Your preferences among ways consistent with your professional standards of increasing practice capacity, such as an additional doctor, more assistants, longer hours, shorter time per patient
- Your interest in a greater range of patient services

Your ODC will need to know your views on basic and personal things that influence the design of the facility, such as:

- Your goals for the practice after five and ten years,
- The point where risk makes you uncomfortable (even when thoroughly researched and organized)
- Your interest in new practice management and marketing techniques to create and cope with accelerated growth in patient numbers)

Your Practice as It Now Functions

The ODC's information-gathering visit gives you a trained observer seeing the normal operation of your practice. Problems you have identified can be verified, analyzed, and considered, and others that seem to merit attention might be noticed.

An appropriately experienced ODC should recognize things such as the causes of a bottleneck, visual or auditory evidence that is creating negative perceptions, or the absence of easily installed evidence that would create positive perceptions. These problems or omissions, and other kinds of opportunities, could be things so familiar to you and your staff that they are as accepted and unnoticed as the paint on the wall. Similarly, during this visit the ODC should be able to notice inefficiencies that may also be too familiar to be noticed by you and your staff. This should particularly include problems that can be solved or reduced by a design change.

ODC time with your staff, especially those with you the longest, should be valuable to your planning. Friendly, not prying conversations with them could help the ODC recognize problems and/or inefficiencies, some of which might be relieved or cured by a better layout.

These discussions can also reveal how your staff feel about the way things are presently done in the practice. These could then be discussed with you, to learn which are considered untouchable, and which you might want to consider changing.

The Conceptual Design Process

The design mission starts with the first steps in the conceptual design process. Your ODC now concentrates more on designing, and less on consulting. By understanding the scope of the conceptual design process you should find it easier to judge whether the visit is a wise investment.

The Conceptual Design Process Steps, Briefly Described

In the conceptual design process steps list that follows, an asterisk (*) marks those that are likely to benefit most from the "face to

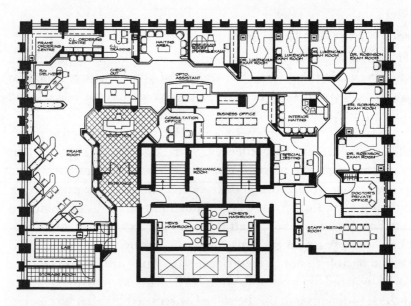

Figure 11–3   Relocation of busy practice into 4,528 sq. ft. on an upper floor of a commanding downtown high-rise office building where they had practiced for years. The space had to go around the elevator core and yield strong appearance, functional soundness, and sense of excellence. (Reprinted with permission from Drs. W. Bruce Robinson and Darcy Lukenchuk, Saskatoon, Saskatchewan. Population 180,000.)

face" visit. A double asterisk (**) identifies others that *might* need to be attempted during the visit (if immediate information is needed).

*1. *Information gathering.* As described earlier.

*2. *Listing design criteria per function.* This detailed and demanding process is discussed thoroughly in Chapters 5 through 9.

*3. *Measuring space chosen or proposed.* This may be needed unless reliable, usually recent drawings of it are available, as with a new building. (Your designer might need a helper to assist in taking the measurements.)

*4. *Opinions of project's operational feasibility.* Based on experience, your designer should ask questions about the planning of your operations and, depending on your replies, make suggestions, give a reliable opinion of feasibility, etc. For example, "How many patients do you want to be able to serve per day in the new office? What operational changes are you considering to increase the capacity of each patient-service and management function, to serve those patient numbers? How do you plan to get the necessary increase in income from the main operations of the practice?"

You may ask the designer, "Will my budget limit permit my project to be built to the size and standards I want?" Equally urgent questions for your OMMC are: "If the budget seems inadequate for the operation wanted/needed, can and/or should it be expanded? What could be done that would justify a higher budget?"

*5. *Budget: Approximate cost range of alternatives.* Building costs should be known to this designer, so the cost of alternatives can be discussed during the visit. These cost figures would be informed guesstimates of the span of cost-per-square-foot for each project version that seems capable of winning your objectives and fulfilling your design criteria.

**6. *Making a conceptual design aimed at your budget target.* If you and your designer agree that it is urgently needed, your designer might tackle it alone that evening, after your meeting. Remember that this will be a *first conceptual design* *plan* based on your objectives, criteria, and targeted budget—not a final design and definitely not a set of working drawings. Although it will be detailed and to scale, it is no more than a first (probably good) suggestion. It couldn't give a contractor nearly enough information for a firm quotation or construction.

7. *Your response to the initial conceptual plan.* This is your evaluation of it after studying it thoroughly and discussing it with any trusted people who know your practice and are competent in your opinion to advise you on this kind of project (your OMMC, your key staff, certain colleagues, a contractor, etc.). This thorough study usually takes a few days or longer, so it is almost never done during the visit. It yields a list of your satisfactions, dissatisfactions, and new ideas that you review with your designer, usually by phone. During that call, have your conceptual plan and covering notes in front of you, for use in discussions. Then, identify what you feel needs to be different, and any new ideas for possible inclusion that you want to introduce, discuss, and/or recommend. During this phone call, your designer should be looking at your plan, and perhaps both sketching and making notes on it.

If you have no suggested solution, your designer should welcome and address it in a positive and creative way.

Your designer may explain why some of the items you want changed are designed as they are, and why they might deserve to remain that way. The choice should then be yours.

If your designer charges a flat fee or a percentage of project cost, there should usually be no additional fee for design modifications, since they are a normal part of the conceptual design process.

**8. *Budget: Guesstimating the cost of the plan.* From knowledge of the current approximate cost of each trade and the materials for building an eye-care doctor's office, your designer should be able to assemble a useful guesstimate of your cost to build the facility shown in this conceptual plan. This guesstimating might be done during the visit, if your designer has brought along current construction cost schedules.

9. *Design revisions to get cost close to budget.* In order to meet your needs and wants (design criteria), and despite your designer's efforts to keep the cost of your initial conceptual design close to budget, cost may be driven above budget (sometimes substantially). When or if that happens, you and your designer will look for items in the design and/or materials that can be revised or omitted to bring down the cost. Although this step is being described at this point in the process, it is almost always taken after contractors have quoted firm prices (the cost is pinned down).

Give yourself adequate time for this soul-searching process. You will usually find it hard to give up things you know are justified, or perhaps just wanted a lot.

You and your designer will propose ideas for cost reduction. After considering them together, you alone choose the deletions you are willing to make. After further thought, you will often decide that some deletions are unacceptable, so those items will be restored, despite the higher cost.

10. *Revised or new conceptual design plan.* An altered or new version of the initial conceptual design plan is prepared in response to your phone call that detailed the changes and new things you want in your facility, the revisions you chose for cost reduction, etc.

11. *Repeating steps 7 through 9.* After you receive the modified or entirely new design, you thoroughly study and evaluate it so you can again tell your designer of any further problems you have identified, recommendations you want to make, and/or new ideas you want included.

You already know that cost and space may prevent your having everything you hoped for in your new facility. Unavoidable compromises should be expected from the start. Choose those compromises carefully, preferably after talking them over with at least your designer and OMMC.

12. *Realistic cost guesstimates for the approved design.* As noted above, your designer should know the current costs of building trades, materials, and fixtures for your kind of project, to give you a useful guesstimate of the total cost of the

approved conceptual design. It has to be a "guesstimate," because an accurate quotation requires analysis of the detailed working drawings and schedules, which is how a general contractor assembles a contract bid.

13. *Your final conceptual design approval.* This will occur when you, your designer, and perhaps your OMMC agree that the latest modified conceptual design offers the best compromises. This is usually not as difficult as you might expect, because the designer's experience should get you at least very close to the best compromise after just a few revised plans. You will be relieved to know that the design is not considered locked up until the working drawings (the next big step) are fairly well advanced.

14. *Renderings (color depictions).* Frequently wanted on big projects (new building, new front on an existing building, an

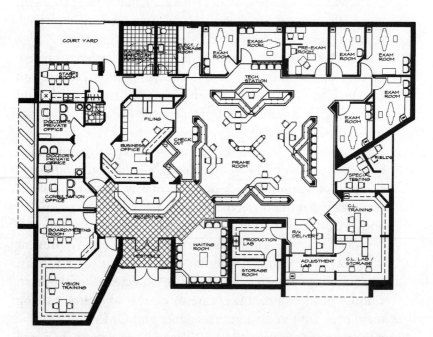

Figure 11–4 Relocation of a busy practice to much bigger, more effective 6,399 sq. ft. space of former bank. As almost always, design was controlled by the doctors' objectives, needs, wants, and ideas. (Reprinted with permission from Drs. Donald Hembree and John Slider, Odessa, Texas. Population 90,000.)

interior view, etc.), these are now often produced by a computer (formerly and still available from artists). Renderings surpass front elevations to show you how it will look. They can require an additional design fee.

Using Other Doctors' Designs for Your Designing

As a source of ideas, the design plans (conceptual designs) of other doctors can often be useful. Getting ideas of "what I would like to have," and equally "what I wouldn't like to have" is important in predesign planning. Look at plans and other offices to get this kind of information, but keep in mind that this potentially valuable move can almost never be a successful substitute for the services of a qualified designer.

To clarify this, compare the question "Can a doctor design an outstandingly effective office as a result of using an eye-care office for quite a few years?" with a question on more familiar ground. "Can a patient, after wearing glasses for quite a few years, select the best lenses needed without having them professionally prescribed?" Surely the answer in both cases is "very rarely."

Since responding to individual differences is bedrock to the planning/designing process, if you obtain other previous office designs as a basis for your design, you will face the risk of getting seriously inadequate information: you will be seeing another doctor's choice of compromises, based on his/her values and circumstances, that could be entirely different from yours.

Also bear in mind that plans showing what was done in projects over the past five to ten years will be illustrating past needs and solutions. You might be unwise to follow yesterday's planning and designing as it was used to meet yesterday's problems and opportunities. Further, since ophthalmology and optometry practice methods are now changing more and faster than perhaps ever before, there is an even greater risk in taking guidance from previous plans.

Aside from probable design weaknesses, when you bypass the services of a designer, you give up the strengths of having your designer representing your interests with your contractor, vendors, etc. This can result in costs that can greatly exceed the amount of the designer's fee.

As expanded below, you almost certainly already know that a *design plan* will never be useable or wanted by a contractor for quotation or construction, as both require a proper set of working drawings. Without these drawings, neither you nor the contractor has control over the cost or what you get.

If you choose to use another doctor's plan, don't overlook the legal point that designs are almost always copyrighted, which firmly establishes who owns them. The use of a copyrighted plan without the owner's permission is illegal.

Since there is no formula for the design of any grouping of eye doctors' offices that might be revealed in their plans, a designer for the process will be a sound investment.

I hope that the foregoing has made the point that the services of a designer and a proper set of working drawings and schedules fills a valid, truly important need and are much to your benefit, even when you are working with the most trustworthy, skilled contractor.

Working Drawings and Schedules Process

The number of sheets and the page titles in a set of "working drawings and schedules" reveal that this, too, is a multistep process. A set may contain many more drawings and schedules than you expect, unless you have experience in major construction projects.

Be sure you fully understand working drawing details, so you can check if you are getting what you want in all the little but important items (e.g., positioning of light switches and electrical outlets). Encourage your designer to explain the drawings in layman's terms. Even after you get the working drawings, minor revisions should be possible, and if unavoidable even a major one (perhaps at extra cost).

The drawings and schedules must be thorough (but don't assume that everything is included), so you, and/or your general contractor will have little trouble doing the following:

- A contractor can make a firm quotation for the completed job as specified.
- You (perhaps with your designer) can control the cost and construction to verify that you get what the contract specifies.
- You can obtain building permits.
- You can obtain landlord approval, when needed.
- You can compile a reliable deficiencies list when construction is nearly finished.

Depending on the scope of the job, a set of working drawings and schedules can contain most or all of the components presented below.

Responsibility Schedule

This is a list of items and services identifying who is responsible for providing and paying for each. The list will be dominated by your contractor or contractors but could include your landlord, or sometimes you when, for example, you obtain and pay for display fixtures outside the contract. This responsibility schedule will be particularly important to you in projects involving landlord participation or more than one contractor.

Design Plan

The design plan is the final version of the conceptual design that you and your designer previously agreed is the best compromise.

The design plan included here likely won't have the notes your designer probably wrote on your prior conceptual design plans, because as one of a set of a working drawings, all explanations needed by contractors (for quotation, construction, or materials procurement), should be available in the rest of the working drawings and schedules.

Partition Plan

This plan looks a lot like the preceding design plan but should show (or indicate where to find) all partition specifications, including height, material (with its rating for sound insulation), fire insulation (sometimes to comply with building codes), etc.

Partitions requiring maximum sound insulation go above or through the ceiling. Still others may be seven feet high, or fence height (30 to 36 inches) to yield an open look while dividing the space.

If any partitions are to function as storage cupboards (perhaps with counters), this will be indicated, but the details will be in "Elevations" and/or "Details and Sections."

This "partition plan" should show the location of the main electric supply panel, and all outlets for: electrical supply, telephones, computers, signal light system, etc. For the location of light switches, see "Reflected Ceiling Plan."

Electrical Schedule

The schedule is a list that identifies all electrical fixtures, their specifications, the manufacturer, the model designation, and the source name and phone number. This schedule will include main electrical supply panel specifications and the required power level (amps) for the project.

Fixture Plan

The fixture plan shows the plan view and location and identifies all cabinetry and plumbing fixtures.

The cabinetry is rarely made on the job, but is more likely fabricated by a remote and sometimes a third-party supplier such as a millwork house (to be good enough to win the right perceptions from your patients and guests). It could include the following:

- Counters, etc., at reception, for checkout and related functions
- Custom-designed side units and other fixtures for the examining rooms
- Work stations throughout the practice (e.g., lens application stations)
- Custom-designed storage units
- Display fixtures of all kinds (in eyewear area, at lens application stations, etc.)
- Privacy cubicles for reception and checkout
- Audiovisual cabinetry for all waiting areas

- Fixtures needed in doctors' offices and the staff/meeting room
- Patient hat and coat storage unit

Other appropriate working drawing pages will show, for each fixture, the elevations, cross sections (as needed), and specifications. Fixtures need to be detailed this well so a millwork house or other source can quote accurately and make them exactly as designed.

The "fixture plan" should show the reference for each fixture (unit identity and page number in the set of working drawings), for finding the drawing and/or details of elevation, cross section and other necessary items, plus the covering specifications.

The design and detail cabinet drawings are there as a description of how the designer wants the fixture to look, and to describe the way it works. A "millwork shop" will produce a set of shop drawings that show how the cabinets are actually made. The designer should review and sign the shop drawings before construction.

Reflected Ceiling Plan

This shows the ceiling for the entire facility, oriented to the floor plan. It should specify the locations and sizes of all light fixtures, air conditioning and ventilating diffusers, and air return grills, as well as the size and arrangement of ceiling tiles. This plan should also show the location of all light switches and which light(s) each switch controls.

Elevations

These pages might not have all the elevations. Some might be scattered in blank spaces on other pages or be absent, depending on how many items and which ones must be specified in this way, and the space available on drawing pages. As mentioned above, each elevation should have a reference designation as on the fixture plan, for ease in finding the other drawing of the item. The detailed specifications for color, finishes, hardware, etc., should be in the "finishing schedule."

Besides providing specifications to all who need them, elevations can present a helpful partial visualization of the fixture's frontal appearance. A rendering, which is more costly, or a photo if available from your designer will be much better at showing you the item.

Fixture Details and Sections

The number of these pages will vary and could be in random locations among the working drawings, on the same basis as the elevations. When your designer knows (from experience) that particular items need to be specified so they will be made as wanted, then details and perhaps cross sections are given. These items can include drawers, cubbyholes, file holders on examination room doors, etc.

A contractor may suggest that you save money on some item by designing it differently. That advice could be correct. However, before ordering any significant change, *always* talk to your designer about which alternative will be best for you. A reputable designer will give you an objective, nondefensive answer, as another normal and important part of professional responsibility (just as you do as a doctor, when you are advising a patient).

Schedule of Finishes and Colors

This schedule identifies the kinds of finishes and/or colors for all items in the design that need these specifications. This should include carpeting, wall coverings, floor tiles, acoustic ceiling tiles, paint, wood stains and finishes, etc. In all cases, the manufacturer's name, product designation, supplier name, and phone number should be given.

If problems of delivery or availability occur, your designer should be able to recommend a suitable alternative and/or to comment on the advisability of one suggested to you by a third person. When an alternative is necessary, this would assure you of getting a substitute that meets all the important specifications. You may risk immediate or future disappointment when someone unfamiliar with the objectives of your project tries to save you money by directing you to a lower performing product, such as carpet that wears out too soon, is recognizably low quality, or is not appropriate for color or texture.

For the specifying or recommending of items or materials, you may prefer to use a designer and/or contractor who is not a supplier of the products involved. Designers associated with or employed by suppliers may of course be talented, independent-minded professionals, but the objectivity of their advice might be reduced by their supplier–employer's interest in selling the products they make or inventory.

Exterior and Interior Signs

Signs need to be effective, and suitable for a doctor's office. Like everything else in the design, they should do their job and cost no more than necessary. You may want your designer to recommend on the basis of experience: kind of sign, size, appearance (typeface style, boldness, etc.), color, lighting, and perhaps the wording. If you are attracted to the idea of a logo, a designer talented and experienced in graphic design could be the right person to design it. When you and your designer have settled the details, these signs should be specified in the working drawings, for the usual purposes.

Graphics

Graphics (in photographic form) have already been discussed at length in the sections on feature displays in Chapter 7. Because graphics such as artwork, photographs, and cartoons can be superior, subliminal ways of communicating, they seem to be growing in popularity in eye doctors' offices.

Graphics can be key contributors to your success by being highly effective in telling a story, and winning wanted perceptions throughout your office (eyewear area, eyewear delivery area, contact lens pod, and interior and main patient waiting areas). If you want to use graphics for any functions in your new facility, tell your designer so locations and space can be planned.

Graphics are almost always used inside rather than outside an eye doctor's office, although a logo should be used in both places. Their locations and specifications should appear in your working drawings. With backlighted transparencies, the design details and electrical specs of the necessary light boxes should be given.

Properly planned locations for graphics will yield a far better result than what happens too often, when graphics such as easel stand pictures from suppliers (if they are good enough to be displayed at all) have no appropriate assigned position and are placed randomly on counters and the floor.

The workup of graphics in your planning and working drawings is the same as for signs (discussed above), but the potential impact and different function of graphics suggests that the choices of location, size, and then the graphics themselves should be done at least as carefully. If one of your team of designers and OMMC is qualified to do so, you may want to use her/him in developing your graphics program.

Mechanical

When these skills are needed, as with the design of an HVAC (heating, ventilating, and air conditioning) system for a new building, or expansion of system capacity in an existing building, these mechanical design drawings and schedules should be produced by specialized professional engineers, whose plans should specify the size of the air conditioning/ventilating unit needed, the sizes of all ducts, and all other technical details.

Some design firms may have "in-house" specialized services of this kind. Others will have an established connection with a reputable HVAC engineering firm.

The Importance of Working Drawings

Working drawings protect *you*, in all that you must expect for your investment. They clarify the responsibilities of all project participants, for their guidance and yours—and for a possible third party (a judge) if you face legal action, such as for noncompliance with a building regulation or local by-law, or some unresolvable difference with a supplier or your contractor.

Working drawings should almost always be used, even for a relatively small construction project, including a startup practice. Almost all contractors prefer working drawings, because they define the scope of work on which they have quoted. "If it's not in the drawings, it's not in the quote." Contractors, quite understandably, don't want to hear, "You should have known I needed this."

Alternatives to Working Drawings

If you are convinced that it will be feasible, and you want your project done without working drawings and schedules, you will need a suitable alternative.

Without doubt there can be circumstances where a project could be done to a doctor's satisfaction without these drawings and their cost. This will be more likely to happen, and perhaps be more feasible (but still not recommended), when the project is relatively small.

You may be tempted to take this route if there are excellent reasons to trust your general contractor for cost, workmanship, timing, and ability to obtain the materials you want. Your confidence would probably be justified if the contractor is a close relative (your spouse, your father, your mother, etc.).

Working without a designer will also be helped a lot if the project site is close to your office, so you can be available often (perhaps several times per day) to answer questions ("What depth are these shelves? How do you want this to look? Will this alternative be acceptable?"). You will need these frequent visits to correct errors before the cost of reversing them gets too high. If you won't be available for these, your contractor will have to decide and then lock things up by proceeding with the work in your absence.

Project Management

When the working drawings and schedules process is completed, you will enter new, critical phases in your project, dealing largely with cost, contracting, supervising, and design.

You may want to use your designer's knowledge and experience by having him/her working for you as an off-the-job "project manager," a normal designer service that clients often use to protect their interests. This can be particularly valuable in the important but probably unfamiliar areas listed and described below.

Put the Job Out to Tender

For public relations reasons (supporting your community) and fast accessibility, you may want a local contractor to quote on and, if feasible, get the job. That contractor might be a friend, an associate (in some other activity), or at least an acquaintance.

There can be a downside to this. Your negotiations before the contract is given and later during construction, and your justified actions to protect your interests, could damage your friendship with the contractor, and the community goodwill you wanted. Your normal desire and actions to get a good job on time and at a fair price could easily bring you more problems than goodwill.

You could shield yourself from the possible negative responses of a local contractor by authorizing your designer to speak for you. Firm stands could then be seen as originating with or at least influenced by the designer.

Further, any contractor, either local or from another area, will recognize (even if they don't like it) that your interests are in the hands of someone whose expertise merits respect. By handling this skillfully with a competent, responsible contractor, your designer should help you get the contracting results you expect, and where a local contractor is on the job, get a reasonable amount of community goodwill.

Often, when working on your quotation, a contractor will phone your designer to get a clarification, ask questions, recommend an alternative, point out an apparent omission, etc. If a bidding contractor comes to *you* with one of these matters, you can point out that it should be referred to your designer, who is your off-the-job project manager. This will reduce both demands on your time, and your responsibility for decisions that could be more serious than they seem.

Also, during the bidding process, your designer, after speaking once or twice with any of the contractors, should usually be able to form a reliable opinion of that contractor's qualifications to undertake your project. This designer opinion should be discussed with you, so you can consider it in deciding which contractor(s) deserve your confidence.

Work with Contractors for Accurate Quotations

Although your designer will usually produce excellent, comprehensive working drawings and schedules, a bidding contractor will almost always have legitimate questions, comments, and suggestions and need additional job site information, etc., in order to be sure that all design details are understood, the design specifies the "best" way of doing things, and there are no serious errors of omission or commission.

These questions and suggestions are signs of a good, conscientious contractor, not a weak one. They are part of the process used by both the contractor and the designer to sharpen the price being quoted, and to get to know and respect each other. If on occasion the contractor brings these items to your attention, they should, as noted above, almost always be referred to your designer.

Contractors know that for their quotation to be accurate, all specifications must be fully understood. Bids based on misunderstood, misinterpreted, or assumed points could be too high or too low.

Too low a bid will rarely help you. It will often spell eventual trouble for you and the contractor. If you accept the bid, the contractor, on finding his/her mistake in the quote, could be forced to choose among asking you for more money, losing money (perhaps a lot), abandoning the job, or even going bankrupt. I have encountered all of those situations, although rarely.

Too high a bid could cause a well-qualified contractor to lose the job, and perhaps cause you to lose a contractor you favor, all because of an honest error in the quote.

If your designer, in answering a bidding contractor's question, can suggest a less costly way of doing something or clarify some potentially costly point, all parties could benefit. Similarly, the contractor should discuss with your designer design points that could, in the contractor's experienced opinion, be specified differently for a lower cost, with equal or better performance.

Even during quotation workup, discussions between the designer and the contractor should be comfortably accepted by both as an act of cooperation for your benefit, not a challenge to either one of them. That way neither side should feel threatened or harassed by the participation of the other.

Analyze Contractor's Cost Breakdown for "Best Value Quotation"

Each contractor should have made a detailed cost breakdown of price per quoted item, which your designer should review to check that each price is close to "best value." To do this, your designer will of course need data (based on experience) on the costs of these trades and materials.

Bidding contractors almost always use a cost breakdown (often called a "quotation breakdown") of trades, materials, and labor to calculate the total price. Your designer should specify that each quotation include the contractor's quotation breakdown so the owner can use it for a better understanding of the quotation and, as seems appropriate, a detailed analysis.

Having each contractor fill out the quotation breakdown form makes a comparison of costs easy and more useful. This breakdown becomes the basis of questions for obtaining the information that ensures an "apples to apples" comparison. Since some contractors are skilled at quoting with intimated inclusions and "not so obvious" exclusions, the time needed to analyze the quotes is well spent.

For your better understanding of this process, a typical quotation breakdown form is shown in Figure 11-5.

Recommend Which Quotations Are Acceptable

Your designer should recommend which bids seem acceptable, and then which one seems best. Although price will be a big factor in the process of identifying the acceptable and best quotations, it should not necessarily control your choice. You will also want to consider other factors that can be imperative in getting for you all critical things you are entitled to from your contractor. The list that follows identifies some of those other things.

- Is the scope of the work well within the contractor's experience-based capacity?
- Will the quality of this contractor's work be likely to satisfy you?

QUOTATION BREAKDOWN

Construction Budget

Doctor_____   Date_____

	Range	Unit Price
		Per Square Foot.
Millwork & Carpentry	$ 15.00 to $ 45.00	$_____
Installation	$ 8.00 to $ 20.00	$_____
Demolition	$ 0.00 to $ 3.00	$_____
Shipping	$ 0.00 to $ 3.00	$_____
Carpet	$ 3.00 to $ 10.00	$_____
Vinyl Flooring & Baseboards	$ 0.00 to $ 1.00	$_____
Electrical	$ 5.00 to $ 26.00	$_____
Drywall	$ 4.00 to $ 8.00	$_____
Ceiling	$ 1.50 to $ 6.50	$_____
Painting, Decor & Vinyl Hanging	$ 1.25 to $ 5.00	$_____
Vinyl Supply	$ 0.00 to $ 2.50	$_____
Aluminum Entrances/Storefronts	$ 0.00 to $ 3.00	$_____
Glass and Mirror	$ 1.75 to $ 6.00	$_____
Signage	$ 0.00 to $ 3.50	$_____
Hardware	$ 0.50 to $1.50	$_____
Quarry Tile/Ceramic Tile	$ 0.00 to $ 5.00	$_____
H.V.A.C. Ductwork	$ 0.00 to $ 3.50	$_____
H.V.A.C. Units (allowance)	$ 0.00 to $ 0.00	$_____

Figure 11–5   Quotation breakdown. One version of a cost breakdown form often used by a contractor and/or designer in calculating a bid or estimate.

Plumbing and Drainage	$ 0.50 to $ 5.00	$_____
Sprinklers	$ 0.00 to $ 2.50	$_____
Display Fixtures	$ 1.50 to $ 3.00	$_____
Blinds/Drapes	$ 0.00 to $ 1.00	$_____
Misc. (Permits, Hoardings, Etc.)	$ 0.50 to $ 1.50	$_____
Structural Work (allowance)	$ 0.00 to $ 0.00	$_____
		$_____
		$_____
	Total	$_____
Gross Area_____Sq. Ft.	@	$_____

Budget Guesstimate is $_____

Budget Range is $_____

ITEMS NOT ALLOWED FOR IN BUDGET -

Designing Fee

Instrumentation

Furniture (Chairs)

Plants

Artwork

Figure 11–5   *(continued)*

- Is this contractor likely to be reliable?
- Is it likely that your job won't be delayed by an avoidable contracting problem?
- Is it likely that the contractor will be able to finance your job with normal advances and payments? Sometimes the designer won't be able to check this.
- Are the payment terms as they should be?

Your designer should tell you about the evidence (both factual and experience-based) that created the impressions behind the recommendation of the successful bidder. When more than one contractor seems acceptable, your designer should suggest a sequence of preference, and if any bids seem unacceptable, tell you why.

You may welcome the responsibility of choosing your contractor, or you may prefer to delegate the choice to your designer (or someone else).

For obvious reasons these recommendations and/or choices should only be made when your designer has no financial or other stake or interest in picking a particular contractor. If there is such a conflict of interest, your designer will usually have made you aware of it in advance and declined making this recommendation. Conversely, the designer, after making you aware of the conflict of interest, might feel free to try persuading you to use her/his associated contractor.

Some design services are linked operations, as in "design–build," where you choose your designer and contractor as a fixed team. "Partnering," another operational option, is not linked since you choose the designer and contractor separately. "Design–build" and "partnering" are discussed in Chapters 12 and 13.

There are many variables. Good advisers, designers, and contractors can be found in quite different settings. There is no formula. So, as always, you must choose carefully.

Review the Construction Contract

Before signing a contract, read it and have it checked by your lawyer.

Add your designer to those reviewing the contract, if that person has, as you would hope, the appropriate experience in checking contracts for projects such as yours. Your designer should be the appropriate person to check that the contract matches the quotation in all construction and materials details, and to easily notice any omissions and/or changes.

Terms dealing with "exclusions" and "qualifications" should be reviewed by your designer, not only to see that they match the quotation, but to make sure you are protected to get all the services and materials specified in your working drawings and schedules.

Your designer should look for omissions of familiar terms that protect you, and the inclusion of any unusual terms that favor the contractor. If these anomalies occur, they should probably be resisted or rejected, as advised by your lawyer.

Also, your designer should identify whether any terms you object to are commonplace in contractors' contracts, so that the contractor would be likely to defend them firmly.

Your qualified advisers should check terms of payment to identify any that are unusual. For example, your holdback payment at the end of construction must be high enough to be effective.

Answer Contractor Questions During Construction

As noted earlier, your contractor should be instructed to go to your designer for all wanted project information, including preparing the quotation, negotiating and concluding the contract, obtaining the materials, doing the demolition (if needed), construction, and millwork.

During construction, there will almost always be necessary and valid questions:

- What is meant here?
- Will this alternative method of construction or material be acceptable?
- How do you want us to respond to this newly found site problem?
- How do you want us to respond to this building inspector's rejection, based on his/her interpretation of the building code?
- Is it OK to make this change needed because a subtrade just found a problem, or because the landlord demands it?
- How should the new idea/change requested by the doctor/owner be handled?

Immediate decisions offer faster action and perhaps lower cost, so you and your contractor will be tempted to make some decisions without consulting your designer. In practice, this occurs fairly frequently, and the results of the action are often satisfactory. Unfortunately, on occasion (which may not be recognized at the time), the consequences impede your objectives slightly, or severely, or even irreversibly (except at prohibitive cost).

An interesting legal question may be involved. If you and your contractor decide to change, omit, or add things and your designer is not included in the consultation, will he/she still be responsible to you when an unwelcome result occurs?

Further, decisions made without the designer can result in a contractor invoice price far above contract price because you approved changes, unaware that you were "ordering extras." One doctor, understandably in a hurry to get into his new office, confidently OK'd many things suggested by his contractor. His invoice price was out-of-sight over the contract price. The contractor explained that the doctor drove up the price by ordering so many changes and extras.

Project control that you wanted securely in your hands or at least those of your designer could be reduced or even lost as a result of this tempting path (tempting because decisions are faster). You may have chosen your designer expecting the safety of project control in your hands and your designer's. For that to happen, you must include your designer in decisions.

If your contractor is reluctant to involve your designer in any questions or suggestions, phone the designer yourself, after telling your contractor, "I'll answer after I've talked with my designer." This will cost clinic time and a long-distance call. That cost will usually be more than offset by what you save from avoiding reduced control over the job and its cost, and likely most important, by lowering your possible disappointment with the results of your venture.

None of the above is intended to suggest that in general, contractors should not be entrusted with guarding and enhancing your interests by obtaining for you, through the high standards of their conduct and work, the project benefits you want. Nor should anything here suggest that the contractor's role in the success of your project needs to be anything but central.

The above emphasis on awareness, control, and careful decision-making is presented to deliver a rightful reminder that when a project must win strong, critically important, targeted results, and also costs a lot of money, you should, and without doubt will want to protect your interests diligently, while still enjoying working with people you can respect, trust, and like.

Make, Negotiate, and See to Final Deficiency List

There are almost always some deficiencies. For example:

1. Items where workmanship isn't up to specified or acceptable standards
2. Incorrect installations, such as wrong fixtures, wrong materials, wrong locations, wrong finishes and/or colors, errors in millwork
3. Errors from incorrect interpretation of working drawings

Although some deficiencies could be serious in their impact on your project's objectives, some might make little difference there.

Construction contract payment terms should call for a holdback amount, paid only after you are satisfied that the project has been completed to the requirements of the contract. That negotiated holdback amount should be substantial enough to be effective if the contractor judges a job deficiency too costly to correct.

The contract holdback is there to protect you in case the contractor fails to pay the subtrades, which would then usually attach a lien to your project. The holdback gives you control of the money to clear liens. Discuss this with your lawyer.

If the holdback amount is near or lower than the cost of correcting the deficiencies, your contractor could (though this is unlikely) be tempted to abandon the job, thus giving up the holdback payment. You would then have the option of a lawsuit, which might not be acceptable to you or might be useless if the contractor's assets are too small.

You will without doubt notice things about the job that bother you, which you will put on your deficiencies list. Your staff will probably point out others. It may surprise you that your designer will probably find more deficiencies than were noticed by you and your staff. Your designer's familiarity with your project's specifications and schedules, and with the process of verifying that the almost-finished job matches them, should make it easy for her/him to notice deficiencies and assemble a comprehensive and reliable list.

After completing the inspection and the list, your designer should give copies of it first to you, and then to your general contractor.

Your designer's inspection for deficiencies will of course require a site visit, perhaps the second, and normally the last at your expense. It should be the final designer responsibility in the project management process. It should include:

- A thorough inspection for and list of deficiencies
- A review with you of the priorities of the corrections needed
- Negotiation with your contractor about the handling of deficiency corrections

You will know which deficiencies bother you the most. Your designer should advise which deficiencies he/she judges will threaten attainment of your objectives, and which if any, are likely to be so costly to correct that your contractor might be very hard pressed.

Your designer should discuss with you whether these more-costly-to-correct deficiencies are important enough to your success (rather than an annoyance) that you should pursue them vigorously. There is an alternative. You could authorize your designer to explore with and assist your contractor in finding less costly approaches than full correction, to minimize the annoyance or damage from that deficiency.

You have every right to insist on a full correction rather than a minimization, but a court case could involve delays, costs (including your time), and risks, such as the rare but real possibility of losing the case or, the contractor not having sufficient assets to compensate you after you won. Your designer might find an acceptable compromise. Although I haven't heard of a court case over deficiencies (they may be rare), and therefore can't report an outcome, some such cases will almost certainly have occurred.

Serious disagreements about the correction of deficiencies between you and your contractor are unlikely. Your contractor will almost always want to please and satisfy you, and will usually find a way of tackling the deficiency corrections that is acceptable to you. But, before you make your final payment, be sure that all the deficiencies that the contractor agreed to correct or minimize have been dealt with.

During the designer's "deficiencies visit," have an agenda of other project matters that concern and/or interest you, and make time to discuss them.

It Is Your Design

Planning and then designing an office with your designer needs to be and almost always is individualized to you. The designer must respond to all your project's givens such as space, financing, kind of community location, and all your requirements and interests, such as your objectives, design criteria (your needs and wants), and your mode of practice. Planning and then designing how the office is to work, such as the proportion of space allotted to the various functions, the "flow," any special design challenges (combining two successful practices, present space to be enlarged)—all need to be individualized to your project.

For a design to be yours, your designer must know you well, your practice, your ambitions, etc., and recognize that your targeted needs, wants, and expectations from your new design should dominate and be respected by all involved through all steps in the project.

From the start, the designer and the others must understand unmistakably that you call the shots in planning your office and its design:

- It's *your* money (the basic, commanding reason).
- The resulting office will be central to your success in reaching *your* goals for *your* practice as a result of *your* project.

Other important to critical reasons will play a part, such as your management and marketing programs, your financial position, your point of view on many of the functions of your practice, and your forecasts of your future needs.

Conversely, a design process that applies a kind of formula aimed at generalized results, or is a designer's idea of what you should want, could be a little or a lot different from what you *do* want, and it puts you on the sidelines.

You will almost always want/expect to control the planning, designing, and building of your facility unless you are working with the Frank Lloyd Wright of eye-doctor office designing, when with your blessing the designer would probably take command. Your designer's role and services in your project (supported by appropriate skills and qualities) must be clearly understood in advance.

For this and other vital designer function reasons, try to have the most promising prospective designer(s) visit you before you are committed to working together. This designer should understand in advance:

- The fact that you are in charge
- The kind of professional relationship you want
- The scope of the designer services you want

The Roles of You and Your Designer, with You in Charge

For you to remain in charge, your designer should be an adviser and resource person, not a decision maker. You will make the choices:

- The project priorities
- Budget, usually a critical factor in most designs
- The look, sequence, and flow of practice services and functions
- How each function will be organized
- What design and contracting services, items, etc., should be included and omitted

For you to be the results-directed decision maker in the design process, you will need to be well informed about the possible reasons why one choice may be better for you than another. Sources of that information include colleagues, OMMC's, ODC's, this book, other publications, and more.

You Could Give Operational Control to an Emissary

If you prefer to reduce or minimize your participation in planning, designing, and installing your project (to devote your time to your practice, etc.), give authority to a senior trusted staff person or family member who is capable of being your emissary.

When the Designer Wants to Be In Control

Since most eye doctors want an excellent income, a designer/consultant may assume that all doctors want their project to bring an annual gross income well over seven figures as quickly as possible. This designer could contend that to be assured of this result, doctors should (must?) defer to his/her "formula that works" and follow all the steps in his/her operating concepts and design. The designer in effect takes control.

This designer might point out that letting her/him take control will be the fastest and therefore least costly way of doing a design and/or the complete project. This could be true, but could also prevent you from achieving some of your objectives. To learn why your control will usually be to your big advantage, check with colleagues about their choices in objectives, practice operation, functional techniques, etc., and their design to accommodate them.

Your Designer as Resource Person, Consultant, and Designer

Other eye doctors, including many with a strong desire to maximize income, will be less comfortable putting the designer–consultant team in command, even if the team leader insists that "for you to achieve your big income target, I must call the shots."

If you are less comfortable giving up control, you will want a designer–consultant who prefers to provide knowledge and experience-based advice and ideas directed by your views of your best interests. Such a team usually responds to your input with a proposed first conceptual design that, as explained elsewhere, is for your criticisms and further suggestions. The conceptual design is then another step in working through the design process with you, not a presentation of what your design should be.

Designs done this way would be as different from each other as the owner/doctors want them to be. Your design would be distinctively *yours* first, then your designer's.

This offers you a serious advantage. Marketing your distinctiveness should contribute powerfully to building your practice and distancing yourself from competition.

Your Ongoing Connection with Your Designer

Things will come up over the months and years in your new facility that you would like to discuss with this designer who now knows you, your practice and your facility so well. Your designer should welcome any opportunity to hear from you and get your news. She/he should also be happy to help you by answering your questions, trying to provide advice, and generally assisting you. Unless it is something big, requiring considerable time, this should be done without charge, and without regard for how often you call.

Your designer should, and surely will, always want you to be aware of his/her ongoing interest in your success and your project.

Flow Chart: The Design Process

The "design process" is a major component in the planning and installing of an eye doctor's new office. It is the subject of a two-page flow chart in Figure 11-6.

An overview of the design process steps usually considered essential, and a common sequence provides both a checklist, and a better understanding of the scope of the undertaking. Bear in mind the familiar caution that although this flow chart covers the important steps in the design process, it presents only one of many possible methods. It is good, but it cannot be taken as standard, since no standard exists.

The first item "Designer's Responsibilities," would have been more inclusive if it presented deserved data on the roles of the other participants taking or sharing responsibility. This was omitted only because the flow chart is already two pages long.

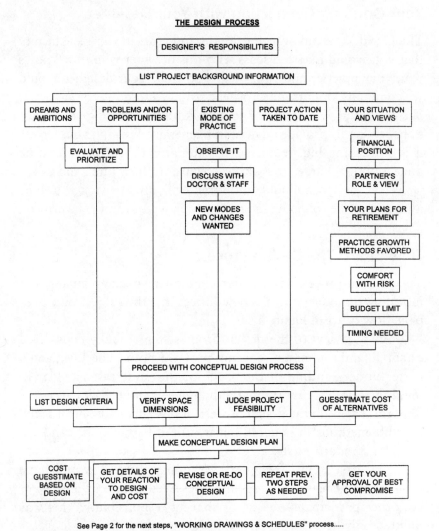

THE DESIGN PROCESS

DESIGNER'S RESPONSIBILITIES

LIST PROJECT BACKGROUND INFORMATION

DREAMS AND AMBITIONS | PROBLEMS AND/OR OPPORTUNITIES | EXISTING MODE OF PRACTICE | PROJECT ACTION TAKEN TO DATE | YOUR SITUATION AND VIEWS

EVALUATE AND PRIORITIZE

OBSERVE IT

DISCUSS WITH DOCTOR & STAFF

NEW MODES AND CHANGES WANTED

FINANCIAL POSITION

PARTNER'S ROLE & VIEW

YOUR PLANS FOR RETIREMENT

PRACTICE GROWTH METHODS FAVORED

COMFORT WITH RISK

BUDGET LIMIT

TIMING NEEDED

PROCEED WITH CONCEPTUAL DESIGN PROCESS

LIST DESIGN CRITERIA | VERIFY SPACE DIMENSIONS | JUDGE PROJECT FEASIBILITY | GUESSTIMATE COST OF ALTERNATIVES

MAKE CONCEPTUAL DESIGN PLAN

COST GUESSTIMATE BASED ON DESIGN | GET DETAILS OF YOUR REACTION TO DESIGN AND COST | REVISE OR RE-DO CONCEPTUAL DESIGN | REPEAT PREV. TWO STEPS AS NEEDED | GET YOUR APPROVAL OF BEST COMPROMISE

See Page 2 for the next steps, "WORKING DRAWINGS & SCHEDULES" process.....

Figure 11–6   The design process.

THE DESIGN PROCESS

WORKING DRAWINGS AND SCHEDULES PROCESS

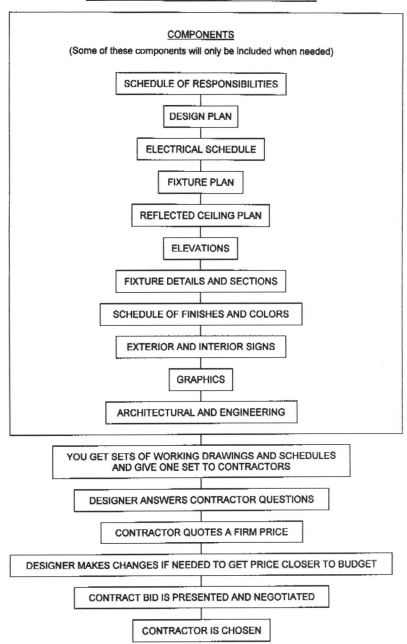

COMPONENTS
(Some of these components will only be included when needed)

SCHEDULE OF RESPONSIBILITIES

DESIGN PLAN

ELECTRICAL SCHEDULE

FIXTURE PLAN

REFLECTED CEILING PLAN

ELEVATIONS

FIXTURE DETAILS AND SECTIONS

SCHEDULE OF FINISHES AND COLORS

EXTERIOR AND INTERIOR SIGNS

GRAPHICS

ARCHITECTURAL AND ENGINEERING

YOU GET SETS OF WORKING DRAWINGS AND SCHEDULES AND GIVE ONE SET TO CONTRACTORS

DESIGNER ANSWERS CONTRACTOR QUESTIONS

CONTRACTOR QUOTES A FIRM PRICE

DESIGNER MAKES CHANGES IF NEEDED TO GET PRICE CLOSER TO BUDGET

CONTRACT BID IS PRESENTED AND NEGOTIATED

CONTRACTOR IS CHOSEN

CHAPTER 12

What to Expect from Your General Contractor

Main Expectations

The functions and level of performance that you should expect from your contractor will depend on what you want, and the services, experience, and dependability offered by that contractor.

There are many sizes and kinds of general contracting operations, and thus a wide range of services available. Their reputations for satisfying their customers can differ significantly. Get references, and a description of each service—particularly their "construction" process, which is usually by far the most costly component of your project.

Your main expectations from your contractor can be reduced to a deceptively short list:

1. Complete the construction job
2. Do it for the least cost, with no hidden or unmentioned costs
3. Do it right
4. Complete it on time

To meet these briefly stated expectations, you will want a general contractor (often called "the general") with considerable experience and ability in:

- Cost control
- Quality control

- Building techniques
- Availability and reputation of subtrades
- Handling of changes
- Communication and cooperation with the other key people involved (owner, designer, project manager, subcontractors, building inspectors, etc.)

To this, add personal qualities that match what your patients expect from you:

- Genuine commitment to client satisfaction
- Fine ethics
- Professional pride in high standards

That may sound like a tall order, and you may decide to settle for less. However, high-caliber contractors are available, and because of the large sum of money usually involved, the standards of contractor ethics noted above are highly important to you.

To maximize your chances of getting the results you want and of being comfortable with your general, take the trouble (and have the good luck) to find one with a fine reputation.

Then inform yourself about your general's concerns and develop a reasonable, nonadversarial approach to them. Recognize that in their job, general contractors routinely face uncertainty and threatening situations such as unknown and/or unpredictable situations, competition, and unexpected demands from you, the client, that could convert a profit to a loss.

Contractor problems become yours if they add to your cost, delay completion, introduce deficiencies, etc. With joint understanding, problems are usually resolved in a way satisfactory to you both. However, it is possible that with a more serious problem (one that heavily raises cost), the contractor may want to look after his/her interests first, which could involve an action or omission that has a heavy negative impact on you. So, even with a first-class, dependable contractor, you should be alert in guarding your interests, as with any key service provider.

As noted earlier, your "general" will usually be prompt in telling you about problems or recommendations (which are usually based on your interests). However, you may be told, "This needs your immediate decision, to avoid costly delay," when the cost us actually modest—far less than you could face from making an unfortunate decision.

Job control should be in your hands, but because you, the owner, are unlikely to have the necessary experience, your designer's participation can be valuable. The designer can serve particularly well as a highly knowledgeable source of advice or participation. This will probably tend to work best when the designer works for you alone (independent of the contractor), although "design-build" has advantages also (can cost less). You might also want to have an on-the-job project manager. An ethical contractor should welcome this if it is handled in a reasonable, knowledgeable, and responsible way.

Because you are likely busy with your practice, much construction will be done without your supervision. Visit the site, or have your representative do so, as often as practical. Although you will probably be working with a general you feel you can trust, you will safeguard your interests best by knowing what is happening on the job as much as is feasible for you. This is not a good time to be away on vacation.

A Small Job

Done by a reliable contractor, a small job can be easier than a big one, with fewer headaches, but will rarely be trouble free. On a small job you may want to choose your contractor in the traditional way, after getting quotations based on your designer's working drawings and schedules. After a meeting or two and a reputation check, your choice of successful bidder will usually depend on price and your confidence and trust that this bidder will meet your four expectations listed earlier.

On small jobs, the *traditional tendering method* of working with a general contractor can be effective, but alternative ways (some described later in this chapter) may be as good or better. Also, even on a small job, you may benefit from using your designer to help negotiate the contract, guide you as the job progresses, and help you solve occasional problems as they occur.

A Big Job

A big job gives your "general" greater challenges, requiring the skills and knowledge of greater experience. Find a contractor whose references, photographs, etc., provide convincing evidence of first-rate competence with similar or bigger jobs (ideally, some for eye doctors).

Your general's experience in the construction of eye-doctor facilities and retail stores will be very valuable to you. A small or fledgling contractor (perhaps the lowest bidder) or a friend lacking enough experience could be beyond their depth on your job because of its size.

Contractor estimates or firm quotes (not guesstimates) should be based on first-class working drawings. Timing predictions (always with the disclaimer "if nothing goes wrong") should be based on the right experience. Before making project cost or timing predictions, a contractor should understand that this is not the usual, probably familiar business office, but is an eye doctor's facility containing specialized clinical and dispensing functions. The clinical accommodations needed in an eye doctor's office also differ greatly from those a contractor may know from previously working on a non-eye-care physician's office.

On the clinical side, the eye doctor could require more partitioning and cabinetry, soundproofing, special lighting, special plumbing, window walls along access routes, more assistant work stations, more internal waiting and information locations, etc.

On the eyewear side, a full-service eye doctor's practice includes an eyewear operation, which is an approximate parallel to fashion retailing, with such "nonoffice" things as numerous displays (with special designs, quality, complexity, and millwork-level finishes), plus display lighting with compensating air conditioning, eyewear delivery/adjustment/ repair stations, etc.

There may be a lens application area with specialized fixtures, and/or a lens production lab with its power needs, soundproofing, benches, and storage cabinets.

These eye-doctor needs mustn't be an "after" shock to your contractor, who could then feel very frustrated over being misinformed or made to look foolish or incompetent through not knowing the differences between an eye doctor's office and one that is not for an eye doctor.

Questions to Ask a Contractor You Are Considering

Selecting your contractor from the candidates who are interested and/or look promising should be done thoroughly. Although price will almost always be a big factor, the lowest bid could be contrary to your interests, as could accepting a contractor about whom you know too little.

The answers prospective contractors give to the following list of questions will help you find those more likely to deserve your confidence and be a comfortable fit with you. Include or omit questions on the usual basis of what feels pertinent to you. Although this information gathering could be most effective as an interview, you may prefer to guard your time by having the prospective contractor fill out a questionnaire. Here are the questions:

- How long have you been in this business?
- Have you worked on other projects for eye doctors?
- If "Yes," please give me the names of some recent ones.
- Have you done any jobs about the same size as mine?
- If "Yes," please name some of those clients.
- Do you normally get involved in design?
- If "Yes," what is the scope of your design service and responsibility?
- Do you expect to do the designing?
- Can you work equally well to my advantage with my designer?
- What client services do you offer?
- How much do you charge per service?
- In each of your services, what is my role as owner?
- Do you quote a fixed maximum price for the construction?
- How do you deal with the costs of design changes while building?
- Will you send me a copy of your standard contract form? When?
- What do you do to help me get good value?
- How long will my job take?

- What follow-up service is included after building completion?
- Will you be able to start construction when all preparatory work is done?

Kinds of Working Relationships with Contractors

With bigger ventures such as constructing a building, the project administration can be set up in different ways. The four methods below have many variations. Also, contractors may have different words for and expanded descriptions of these methods.

Traditional Tendering

You are probably familiar with its basics. A designer or architect produces a set of working drawings for each contractor. This is the "bid package," which includes, as needed:

- Design drawings
- Specifications and schedules of materials
- Engineered and electrical plans and specifications
- Mechanical (plumbing, HVAC, sprinklers, etc.) plans and specs
- Structural design plus civil engineering (site work) plans and specs

This "contractor's bid package" contains the needed drawings and specs, plus cost breakdown analysis and contractor instructions. These are sent to the few general contractors you selected because of their reputation and your confidence in them.

Their bids (quotations) are gathered and analyzed. Some items may be questioned and requoted. Each quote must be sufficiently qualified to ensure comparison of "apples to apples." Check that inclusions and deletions don't leave potentially misleading impressions.

The doctor/owner (you) and the designer analyze the quotation summaries, and you choose your general contractor for the project. Your choice will usually be influenced strongly by price, and then the other four basic things you want from your contractor (listed at the start of this chapter). At this time further negotiations often occur, particularly concerning design changes to lower the cost.

The foregoing is a simplified version of the traditional tendering process for a fairly large project. A small project would be simpler, a much larger one more complex. There are many different versions of and variations within this process, but the main points are as above.

Traditional Tendering Positives

- A set of drawings nails down the project as much as reasonably possible.
- You know the real costs.
- You choose your contractor on a researched and competitive basis.

Traditional Tendering Negatives

- The process is adversarial, so each party does what is best for them. Sometimes someone loses. It can easily be you, the owner.
- The general who will be on the job is not connected with the planning process.
- It is late in the process when you find out what your costs will be.
- The up-front time needed for "bid package" thoroughness adds to your cost.
- Cost reduction deletions so late in the process could increase your sense of loss.
- A lengthy time is often required for the process of deleting and amending items to reduce cost.
- Designer, contractor, and your interests can conflict and result in extra costs:
  The *designer* could want advance notice of revisions, or you might be charged for "extras" or "change orders," and you could face additional cost from delays. It is of course impossible to advise the designer about changes before the need for them is recognized.
  The *contractor* could notice things that will be needed in construction and aren't in the drawings, but say nothing and leave it out of the quotation so it can become

an extra, charged separately later. If the item is large,
its exclusion from the price could lower the quotation
enough for that bidder to win the contract. Then, the
item's absence from the quote would permit the contractor to make a big extra charge.

The *client* could want to bypass the designer regarding
changes and make decisions alone with the lowest bidder when a cost-cutting need becomes known late in
the process. The consequent delays will be costly. This
gives an opportunity to the contractor, who may need a
way to make the job profitable or be willing to use this
situation to improve profit.

Also, because you want the job done right and on time with
minimum extras and hassles, you could feel threatened when
unpredicted things threaten these goals. You could thus be open to
making decisions without knowing the cost.

Project Management

This is usually undertaken by another contractor, a skilled, experienced person or company, perhaps specialized in project management, working under contract with you.

The first step is the same as in tendering above. A complete
set of bid-document design drawings is produced by the designer.
The project manager (PM) puts the drawings out to bid with subtrade contractors from each discipline (electricians, plumbers,
etc.), obtains the quotations, analyzes them, and assembles a cost
budget for the project.

The PM runs the job. The PM, sometimes with the owner's
participation, chooses the subtrades and makes an individual contract with each. The PM also obtains the materials and fixtures,
sets and supervises the timing and faithfulness to specification of
the construction, and is on site daily to supervise and coordinate
construction.

There is no total contract price. Your PM makes all cost-
sensitive choices, often for reliability first and then price. Payments
are made to subtrades by the owner through the PM. Project manager fees are commonly a percentage of the actual project cost.

Because you probably lack experience in project contracting of this kind, and because you lose money when not serving patients, project management can be attractive. With the right person or firm, it could be all right. However, your control over price, timing, and satisfaction will be reduced, which could involve too much risk for that hoped-for gain. Think it over carefully.

Since trust is so important when you delegate so much, a suitably experienced family member or close friend (perhaps retired from a successful contracting career) should have the ability and loyalty to you to be a good PM. Otherwise choose on the time honored basis of reputation.

Your designer would often be well qualified as an on-the-job PM, but unless he/she is local and not too busy, travel distance and lack of time would usually make daily supervision unworkable. However, to the considerable extent usually feasible, your designer can be a valuable resource person in off-the-job project management, as suggested in the previous chapter.

Project Management Positives

- The right PM working well with you and the designer reduces the time you must be away from your practice, which improves your financial picture.
- The right PM can effectively control project finances.
- The job is run by an "owner advocate" with no conflicting interests.

Project Management Negatives

- Additional time will be required for the "tender drawings," increasing cost.
- You will have no firm cost for the total job until it is finished.
- Suitable project managers are hard to find.
- Your time to manage the manager will still be significant or you would be delegating protection of your interests to a relatively unsupervised person.
- Your designer will usually not be involved in the inevitable changes (though perhaps still responsible).

Design–Build

As the name implies, an experienced professional designer and suitably qualified construction contractor working together in a single operation, or on some other basis of close association, provide both project design and construction. They may also expect to do your predesign planning, or it might be done by independent consultants, one in design, the other in ophthalmic management and marketing, as described earlier. Check their track record for qualifications and experience with projects for other eye doctors.

On completion of the conceptual design process, they usually quote either a firm figure or, quite often, a "not-to-exceed" amount that gives you an early handle on contracting cost.

They may quote designing and contracting separately, as the cost of the design phase may be your opening commitment. However, the total is almost always the significant figure, as the individual quotes may be adjusted to make the design cost look modest versus competition who are not working in the design–build mode.

The close relationship of the designer and contractor in design–build should offer the advantage of saving you the cost of delays: when the contractor sees a need, he/she can immediately suggest a less costly design option to the design side, or the designer can quickly provides the build side with design or specification changes needed because of unexpected construction problems, needed materials substitutions, your request, etc.

In design–build, the two participants prepare a proposal for you, the owner, which may have an itemized design fee and an outline of how the contract will work. Usually, a fee is quoted for the conceptual design, which should cover an interior and/or exterior design plan. When you accept that fee, the design–build firm usually assembles a "not-to-exceed" budget.

All this gives you, early in the process, a design, an interior and/or exterior look, and a total budget cost to build that design. That construction quote is usually supported by data on the cost components. By accepting this budget quote you will have agreed to retain this design–build operation for your project. You, the owner, then have a realistic budget to obtain the financing, while continuing to give direction on design.

The designer and contractor will both be at management level in their operation, so either should be able to minimize delay in answering your questions, responding to your concerns and/or complaints, acting on your suggestions and requests for changes, etc.

D/B can also be to your disadvantage. When design and contracting are combined in one operation, you have no independent adviser on either the design side (to advise you on a contracting matter) or the build side (to advise you on a design matter). You may want to find independent advice when you need to judge and decide about important matters of project design and contracting.

There is another possible design–build disadvantage. Once the design is agreed and the contract signed, your project knowledge and participation could diminish. Without referring to you, the contractor, the designer, or both could be making important project decisions. However, when your practice gives you very little free time, or when you would rather delegate most project responsibility, you may prefer this, even though when bypassed, you lose some job control.

The design–build team's reputation and desire to do your job, plus your comfort with them and the service they offer, could be pivotal in your decision.

Design–Build Positives

- You have early control over budget and design.
- The project moves faster because of efficient designer–contractor communication.
- If not an illusion, design costs could be lower because of the contractor–designer relationship.
- You will have only two closely associated people to deal with regarding changes and questions.

Design–Build Negatives

- On cost-control deletions and changes, you could be bypassed because the D/B team wants to avoid the cost of delay. You would thus have less or no input in some "cost versus benefit" decisions. You will need to put a high level of trust in the D/B team.

- In the same way, your involvement in and knowledge of job progress or problems could become minimal, reducing your control.
- You will have little or no control or influence over who works on the project because, after setting total cost and completion date, a D/B contractor will probably prefer to focus more on profitability and finishing on time than on responding to you.
- You must accept in advance the designer selected by the contractor, and vice versa.
- The designer, or the contractor, could encounter a conflict of interest with you where a choice must be made between loyalty to you or to the design–build associate. Your interests in this situation that you probably will know nothing about will remain unprotected.

Partnering

Partnering is relatively new in the design–construction field. It is now used in the design and construction of a significant and growing percentage of both private and public projects.

In partnering, a team of the owner as "key player," a designer, and a contractor you have chosen work on the project together, particularly in decision making. As owner, your best choices will usually be a designer with a good track record in eye doctors' offices and retail stores, and a similarly experienced general contractor who knows the local area and has a fine reputation. This, plus a good personal fit among the team members, plus commitment, should provide most of what's needed.

After you have selected your team candidates, you all meet, usually in your office. The expense of bringing the proposed team together will involve a modest outlay (investing a little to protect your big investment). At this first, critical meeting, the three of you discuss and agree on the division of project responsibilities— the "scope of work." This is critical to the process because the designer and contractor quote their respective fees on the basis of their separate responsibilities. If they win your confidence, and their fees are acceptable, they are your team, but perhaps on a probationary basis at this point.

With you and the contractor participating, the designer then goes through the conceptual design process to create a design. On completion of the preliminary design, the contractor and designer determine a project budget. The contractor then quotes a "not-to-exceed" amount for the job. You all then work on the reality of cost goals to finalize the design/budget process. Next, the working drawings and schedules are completed. Then, the project is tendered, and a fixed price is determined from the quotes.

The contractor's fixed price will include a contingency amount, to handle small extras and surprises along the way. There will also usually be a mechanism in the contract to split any unused part of the contingency amount and any savings that this partnering team can produce. This mutual benefit split is an added incentive to the contractor and designer to reduce the project cost.

For changes or cost reductions, the designer, contractor, and you work together to produce and use exact, supported figures for additions and removals. You always participate in the value/priority judgments of change costs versus your benefits. You have final approval of subtrades and costs before the job is started. The usual payment holdbacks, etc., are in the final contract. After completing the assigned duties, the designer stays in touch with the project, as a member of the team.

Your ongoing participation gives you control in matters of cost, timing, quality and effectiveness of the work, etc. Major problems are resolved or reduced by talking them out among the three parties responsible for the project's success. Problems are usually dealt with long before they become large.

You and the other team members may live quite far apart, but this shouldn't be a big handicap as, aside from the first, face-to-face meeting and another near the end of construction, all other meetings involving all three parties can probably be done effectively by phone and e-mail, and the costs should be more than offset by your benefits.

Partnering Positives
Routine timing in design and construction should be good because:

- Budgets are formed early in the process.
- Team decisions and ideas are better and faster with "all-party" consultations.
- Changes are known to the owner and subject to her/his input.
- A less costly minimum (working) drawing design package is appropriate.
- The owner controls design and cost via team members, to best determine value.
- The designer and the contractor tend to be most effective because they work directly with the owner.
- Teamwork reduces the likelihood of shortcuts being unknown to any of the three parties.

Partnering Negatives

- More owner time is required, to keep the process moving.
- This is "leading edge" and therefore relies more on the relationship of the team members than on an established operating formula.
- It doesn't favor speed. When the shortest possible job time is essential, partnering might seem impractical, although it could be no more time consuming than other project methods when those are performed thoroughly.

Owners usually want to be active participants toward the success of their venture. That may explain the popularity of partnering, particularly in big projects where so much is at stake.

Judging Which Method Will Be Best for You

We are aware of design and construction success with each of the above methods. The best method for you will often be determined by:

- Your understanding of and respect and trust for your chosen professionals
- Your view of the benefits and hazards of delegation
- The cost of your time, versus the cost of things you could have been aware of that can (and often do) go wrong

Bids That Are Unusually Low or High

In choosing among contractor bids, widespread experience suggests that you should put aside any noticeably high or low bids. With an unusually low bid you will often end up paying the real job cost, which will tend to be an average of the middle bids. And you of course want to avoid the high bid that is well over the "real" cost. An experienced designer should be able to advise you on bid reality.

Designer and Contractor Duplication of Client-Guidance Services

Some contractors offer client-guidance services that appear similar to those of your designer as described in the preceding chapter. To choose, you will need to know about any differences in these services, to be sure you are comparing apples with apples. This may be confusing. As the owner, you want to be able to choose which will be the most appropriate professional guidance in your planning.

Also, make sure there is no overlap or duplication in services you are contracted to receive from your project participants. Your designer, architect, contractor, etc., should assure you that you won't pay twice for the same thing.

CHAPTER 13

Feasibility: Costing, Financing, and Budgeting a New Office

Venture Analysis

This chapter shows one way you can judge your proposed project's feasibility by analyzing it as a "venture," a business investment.

The Process of Feasibility/Venture Analysis

You have done your homework. You are finally sure that you need a better facility. You have an image of what it should be. Now you need to know:

- How much will it cost?
- Can I find the financing?
- How much can I afford?
- Will it pay enough soon enough to justify itself?
- Am I comfortable with this as a venture?

Feasibility: Costing the Venture

You would never commit to a major purchase or investment without knowing how much it was going to cost. In fact, cost probably controls many of your bigger personal *buying* decisions. The word "buying" is emphasized to remind you again of the pivotal difference between buying and investing.

Investments are usually chosen for their expected return. Therefore, your decision to proceed with this major investment

315

will depend on cost as justified by probable return, and whether your lender agrees.

Project Cost: Who Is Best Qualified to Estimate It?

A designer and/or contractor well experienced in facilities for your profession will usually be best at predicting cost for:

- A new building for your practice
- Installing your practice in an existing space
- A major renovation and/or expansion of your existing office

Project Cost Estimating: What Is Involved?

1. What Your Designer and/or Contractor Need to Know about the Space

- Is it a building to be erected for you only?
- Is it a building to be erected for multiple tenants?
- Is it a condo, to be built or renovated?
- Is it renovation of existing space? In what kind of building?
- Will a landlord or third party be involved in the project specifications, etc.?

2. Expected Interior Contracting Costs

Your designer and/or contractor will probably have constantly updated lists of the approximate cost of interior construction components that go into construction projects. These lists are used routinely to estimate project cost and to help set the price on a formal job quotation. If feasible, see the check list of a local designer and/or contractor, to help you understand the dollar total for your job, and to help you find places where you will accept a lesser item or omit it to reduce cost.

Below is a list of some items common to ophthalmology and optometry practice projects:

- Demolition (removal of existing items)
- Shipping of material or fixtures to the site

- Carpet, hard surface flooring, ceilings, glass (including interior window walls) and mirrors, signs (interior)
- Display fixtures (the cabinetry and hardware needed to hold and present items)
- Air conditioning units, distribution and duct work, adequate to remove heat from eyewear room display lighting, and from the operation of lab machinery (this air conditioning almost always exceeds that needed in a usual business office)
- Draperies or blinds, particularly when needed for your level of light control in window rooms
- Sprinklers
- Cleanup

In addition to the air conditioning, there are two other items that are often more extensive than a contractor would expect in a job described as an "office."

- Electrical, lighting, and wiring for numerous clinical functions, the eyewear area, and the lab are usually absent in other professional or business offices.
- The number of partitions, including those with sound insulation, and the total length of partitioning will exceed what is normal in a usual business office.

A contractor who has given a ballpark estimate (guesstimate) without seeing a design plan and talking to the designer can be forced to substantially amend it on learning that the job is going to cost a lot more than is usually involved in general offices (for accountants, insurance firms, etc.).

3. Expected Exterior Contracting Costs

These costs are also assembled by your designer and/or contractor from lists similar to those used for interior costs. They occur when you buy land, erect a building, or modify an existing building's exterior. Exterior work includes all things that need to be done on:

- The lot
- The foundation
- The outside of the building

4. Lot Development Cost

- Ground water dispersal, with possible holding storage and/or storm sewers
- Adequate parking for long-term needs and local use codes
- Setbacks from street and property lines—these can affect building size and shape
- Location of and ease of access to building services: electrical, water, sewers, etc.
- Soil replacement if lot was previously a service station, chemical plant, refinery, etc.

5. Foundation Cost

This of course only occurs when a building has a basement, not when it is on grade (has a slab). Basement space is sometimes wanted because of its lower cost. A slab is favored if the foundation construction history of the area shows that a basement will cost too much.

6. Building Shell Cost

This will depend on building size and how it is built. Allowing for practice growth, a sole occupancy building for an eye-care practice usually needs 4,000 to 10,000 square feet. A wood-frame or wood-truss building will almost always cost less, because of lower labor cost.

Building materials also affect cost. The popular exterior finishes are wood, vinyl, metal siding, privet, or brick. The cost of some materials, such as brick, varies a lot per location.

7. Unexpected (Nonroutine) Building Costs

Costs that can come as a surprise occur often enough to deserve mention here. Experienced designers and contractors try to protect you and themselves from these sometimes costly surprises, which are illustrated below:

- Electrical service in an existing building (such as an older home) may be inadequate: there may be 30 amp service, when you need 100 or 200 amps.

- The existing heating, ventilating, and air conditioning (HVAC) system may be inadequate.
- Fire separation may be needed in ceiling, floor, demising walls (those to adjoining suites) in order to satisfy local codes and get interior construction permission.
- Exits and means-of-exit must be brought within code for the square footage of office, and handicap accessibility may be more costly than usual, or even too costly.
- Structural analysis may be necessary for a beam needed because load-bearing walls are gone or breached.
- Access to a four-inch sanitary drain with proper venting is needed.
- Existing sprinklers may not meet present code requirements.

8. Cost Cutting Mission Is Normal

You and/or your intended lender may conclude from the feasibility study that the cost is too high. You then look for the least damaging ways of cutting to the level needed.

As discussed earlier, omissions and changes to reduce or try for the lowest cost occur often. This process can and often does lead to the removal of items and a new plan. Then, after study of the new reduced plan, and before construction starts, many doctors ask that some items be put back. This is also normal in designing, as you and your advisers look for the best compromises (to meet all objectives and criteria including cost). But it can produce delays, and these might add to cost.

To minimize the costs of delay, discuss the changes with your designer for experienced guidance before a new plan with your design changes is started, so the changes can be chosen using the best information, and then verified as feasible by all concerned.

Make a prioritized list of needs and wants to guide you. Places to cut cost can also come from the lists of expected construction costs prepared by the designer and contractor.

9. "Ballpark" Guesstimates of Project Costs

Based on projects done in and near the year 2001, here are ballpark guesstimates of costs per square foot to install an operation capable of producing an adequate return on investment:

- A new 3,000 sq. ft. building with complete interior (not including cost of lot or its development): $110.00 to $130.00 per sq. ft.
- Interior only for 3,000 sq. ft.: allow $60.00 to $70.00 per sq. ft.

These figures are presented as a rough guide, to give you some idea of what you could face. Within each year they can go up or down (usually up). Also, there can be considerable local differences in construction costs. For more reliable guesstimates, get advice from appropriate designers and contractors experienced in your profession's facility projects in your area.

Even if you know of projects completed for less than the above, these numbers can be useful as a starting point in guesstimating a project's cost.

Feasibility: Finding Your Financing

Educate Your Banker

Your lender will often be a bank. Remember that in working with a bank, you are in fact working with a *person* who will be making decisions very important to you. Early in your discussions, start a thorough program of educating your banker (this person) about your profession, particularly as you practice it.

If you are an optometrist, it is entirely possible that a banker won't really understand:

- That you are a doctor, a respected health-care professional, not a merchant
- The stature of optometry today, particularly in the United States and Canada
- Your education as an optometrist
- The scope of your total service, including advances coming in optometry

To build your banker's confidence in your optometric venture, take your banker on a tour of an optometric college. Also try to take her/him to at least one colleague with a successful practice similar to your goal.

If you are an ophthalmologist, your banker can be expected to have a better grasp of your operation, but this should be carefully verified when you are applying for financing.

Doctors in both professions should talk often and honestly with their banker and insist that the banker reciprocate. Be sure your banker understands your venture. Build your banker's confidence in you.

Shop Around

You will usually go first to a previous, satisfactory lender. But be ready to find another if it seems needed, or just to protect yourself. Look for the best deal, the most receptive banker. If the banker insists on considering you as a commercial enterprise, look for another banker.

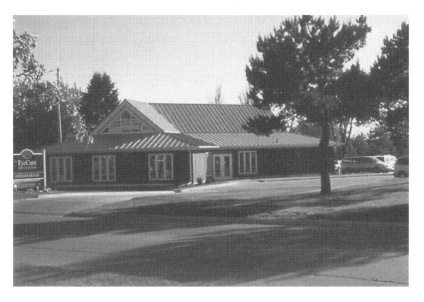

Figure 13–1 To help build lenders' confidence, show a portfolio of interior and exterior photos of your concept, such as this new building designed for two newly joined, expanding optometric practices. (Reprinted with permission from Drs. Steven Boeke and Jerry Stahl, Waterloo, Iowa.)

Show Faith by Committing Your Own Capital

This is critical in winning a lender's support. Not surprisingly, the lender concludes, "If this applicant won't make a significant personal investment, this proposal must be dangerously risky."

If you have little or nothing to invest, the proposal must reflect this by using all feasible ways to hold down the amount to be borrowed. This is a separate subject discussed in Chapter 10, in the section on financing a startup practice.

Your Complete, Impressive Business Plan: Opening Thoughts

Your business plan is usually pivotal in the decision of your lender, and is just as important for your guidance. It needs a good format. The plan could run to twenty pages or more, depending on your proposal's size and complexity. Among other functions, it should reveal to your lender two necessary points: the observable strengths and the potential risks of your planned venture.

Some banks have extensive material to help you develop your plan. Or, you may want help from a financial adviser. If your profession's management consultant and/or your accountant has successful experience with eye-doctor business plans, ask one of them for guidance. It is usually too important to tackle alone.

A Banker's View of the Elements of a
Sound Business Plan for an Eye Doctor's Venture

Because optometry is often less understood by bankers, I decided to ask a well-placed banker who was willing to provide guidance on the writing of an appropriate business plan for an eye doctor's new or remodeled office venture, to direct his attention to that profession. I met with a banker whose management responsibilities included influencing the reworking of policies in the appropriate loans department of his large bank. He agreed to write his ideas for assembling a comprehensive and impressive business plan for an eye-care venture (in this case optometric) and to do it only after informing himself about that profession through the visits suggested earlier. He did a fine job of informing himself, and then assembling his ideas. Most of the preceding "opening thoughts" and the following thirteen-point outline (which I agree with) are his. Much of his advice will also apply to ophthalmologists planning such a venture.

A Banker's Thirteen Elements of a Sound Business Plan

1. *Introductory letter.* This should note briefly the objectives behind your business plan and why you believe they are feasible and worthwhile.
2. *Title page.* Give the practice name (and your name, if it is not that of the practice), practice address, phone number, fax number, your home phone number, and the date.
3. *Table of contents.* This should list all major headings and subheadings in the plan.
4. *Summary statement.* This summary of your proposed venture should include:
   - A description of your practice now
   - A predictive description of your "new practice" after one and five years
   - Projected earnings after one and five years
   - Total money needed, including all debt payment in the first year
   - Security you have to support loan financing
   - How and why you expect increased earnings to pay off loan financing
5. *Background information.* Include your education, credentials, practice startup, success to date, and special recognition professionally or in your community (to reveal your practice to date).
6. *Your profession.* In addition to your lender, other readers of your plan need to know your view of your profession's role in your community, trends in its practice that will probably affect your practice, your competition (now and foreseeable) and its impact on your practice.
7. *Services offered.* Beyond the description of your new practice (item 4, the summary statement), this section should identify the new services you will offer, emphasizing the patient benefits that will help practice building (marketing). List new instruments for all diagnostic and treatment procedures.

8. *Practice building (marketing).*
   - How you plan to attract the additional patients you expect
   - How you expect to get additional income per patient
   - What advantages patient perceptions of you will yield over other local providers
   - Your plans for contacting established patients and the general public in your area
9. *Location, land, building(s), and equipment.* Describe briefly the physical requirements of your new facility and practice, and why you targeted them.
10. *Operations.* To show that you have control over all aspects of your practice, describe:
    - Your human resources plan—the number of full-time and part-time staff you will have, their total remuneration, job descriptions, and reorganization in terms of annual cost
    - Controls over cost of inventory
    - Cost of inventory for all supplies you dispense or consume
11. *References.* This should include lists of:
    - Investors or partners involved now or soon
    - Banks or other financial institutions who lent you money in the past
    - Other doctors with comparable practices who have invested in a similar venture
    - Other doctors with whom you now cooperate
12. *Financial plan.* This should show a potential lender:
    - All capital requirements
    - Annual profit and loss statements for your practice to date
    - Cash flow budgets for the previous year, and one-year projections for the first five years after the project
    - Your personal financial position, including assets and all debts and obligations
13. *Foreseeable risks and problems.* In a worst-case scenario, describe where you would want to avoid or at least minimize the risk and its impact. The bank should view this as an indication of thorough preparation on your part, and of your

troubleshooting ability. If the bank wants to use this worst-case scenario as the basis for your financing, find another bank.

If Your Loan Is Refused

Don't give up. Find out why. Then, if you feel it is worth the effort, make acceptable changes in your proposed venture that address the lender's objections. A refusal is not necessarily final. If you want to continue with this lender, at least so you haven't wasted all the effort you have put into getting financing from them, inform them of your changes and, if it seems needed, improve their familiarity with your practice.

Beyond all this, as a good professional courtesy, return to the banks you have approached, while also taking your proposal to other banks and presenting it to them confidently.

Also, talk to your team of advisers (management consultants, designer, general contractor, etc.), and your colleagues who have completed a project. Sometimes one or more of them will be able to suggest alternative sources of financing.

Feasibility: Budgeting

Your feasibility study should be a sound business analysis of your venture that increases your project control and reduces your risk by improving your probability of success.

To get these benefits you will need a reliable *forecast of additional income*, in order to find your budget limit. When you have your budget limit and reliable estimates of cost, you will be ready to find your financing.

Contributors to Your Investigation

- A suitably experienced designer/consultant with a verifiable track record
- A management/marketing consultant in your profession, also with a track record
- Contractors, particularly those experienced with eye doctors' facilities
- Your accountant

- Colleagues who have done a similar project (they can provide excellent guidance)
- Your spouse and family, who may not have expertise, but are usually loyal allies
- Dedicated staff, with extensive knowledge of your practice, your community, etc.
- Experienced business friends
- Your banker

There will almost certainly be some differences among their recommendations. Whose advice should you use? You will surely favor those whose judgment and experience give you the best sense of reality, and thus confidence.

Growth in Patient Numbers

The average annual increase in patients served per optometric practice in the United States in 1996 was about 50 (about 1 a week). In one of two theoretical examples I used here, I assume forecasted growth figures of 1 to 3 *per day*, and 2.5 through 4. In a 245 working-day year, 1 per day is 245 additional patients per year, and 4 per day is 980, or 5 to 19 times that in the 1996 AOA survey.

When considered against the one percent national population growth, and the 800 new practitioners in that year (1,150 graduates less 350 retirees), the increases in the rate of growth of patient numbers that I assumed for the examples seem highly unlikely, although those figures should be improving now because of the aging population and the lessening unpopularity of glasses.

From analysis of statistical data authoritatively processed from survey evidence, the AOA concluded that it cannot be assumed that masses of patients are waiting to be served. In view of this statistical data, how does one explain *some* eye doctors' reports of much higher than usual practice growth after moving into a new, stronger facility? The answer: evidence and common sense urge that the facility made an important contribution, but it is equally evident that these eye doctors were already doing and continued to do a lot of things right in their practice, and that they did a fine job of planning and executing their ventures. For example, they probably improved their practice marketing. At the same time, evidence and common sense urge that the facility made an important contribution.

I have no statistical, survey-based data to support the assumed, seemingly unlikely growth forecasts that are strongly attributed to an impressive new facility. My evidence is anecdotal, without numbers. Despite that, I believe the assumed growth numbers are a realistic conclusion to infer from these success stories. Some practices, after moving to a much superior facility (and possibly a better location) have reported satisfaction that must have involved those assumed rates of growth.

One such anecdote illustrates the point. A successful ophthalmology practice in a modest-sized U.S. prairie city had reached capacity, even though a relatively new ophthalmology practice in town was doing well, a big "advertising" chain had more recently opened, and there were other eye-care practices in town. Eye-care service seemed abundant. While discussing proposed expansion, the already highly successful doctor/owner asked me, "Where will the additional patients come from?" I could only answer that I had some ideas about it, but no firm answers—but if demographics controlled it, why was he now at capacity despite the new competition? He didn't have an answer. The doctor doubled the size of his facility and made substantial improvements to his operation. I am told that he is thoroughly pleased with the results.

Surely the most important question is whether the additional patients and income *will* come. You will need to investigate and weigh the anecdotal evidence against any opposing demographics data. Then decide on the likely impact of each on the growth of your practice and income.

Try to learn from colleagues who completed an observably successful project, if the fixed factors (economics of the area, location, competition, etc.) where the practice is located match yours, and whether the controllable ones (strength of the new facility, practice marketing program, etc.) seem apt to work for you.

There can be quite a few reasons why, after the change, patients come in more often, and strangers choose to come. The main reasons (some mentioned previously) seem to be that:

- The facility wins the right perceptions both outside and in
- New surgical techniques for vision correction
- A new marketing program is much more effective
- Patients derive a feeling of possible advantage from going to such a successful doctor
- Excellent announcements stimulate interest (act like recalls)
- Reluctance to wear glasses diminishes, because a place this attractive "may help me look the way I want"
- A feeling of prestige comes from going to *the best*, the place people are talking about
- People want to be one of those who knows all about this new operation
- For established patients, the promise of new, more appealing eyewear leads to a return visit far sooner than usual
- Interest grows in the benefits of superior performance lenses
- The enthusiasm of existing patients for your new facility wins referrals

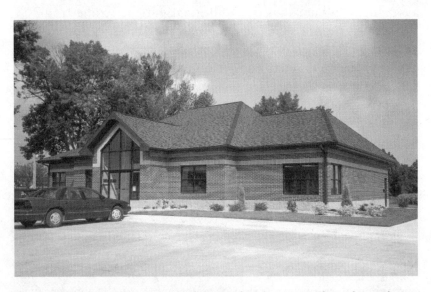

Figure 13-2   To add to your confidence that forecasts of accelerated practice growth are realistic, examine photos such as this, and as feasible visit the new facilities of colleagues. (Reprinted with permission from Dr. Craig Semler, Hampton Iowa.)

Even though the excellent contribution of an eye doctor's facility to the practice rate of growth is clearly evident (and still seriously neglected), it is only one of the powerful factors involved. The foregoing may help to explain the reported success stories. Your only method of checking will be that constantly repeated point: see, or at least talk to your colleagues who have had the experience. Also, see the "colleague survey report" in Chapter 14.

Because of these observable stories of success in spite of the statistical data you will want a reassuring way of choosing which evidence to use. I suggest that you accept both, based on the obvious existence of exceptions to the general picture.

As noted in the next section, you will want to explore your project's feasibility by analyzing practice numbers that are as close to your reality as your history, and evidence from statistics and colleagues permits.

Reality in Figures and Calculations

The reliability of your planning improves when you use actual (perhaps your own) numbers or at least realistic ones in your feasibility study. Forecast your growth after considering reports from colleagues. Their figures can help, but not if you feel that they are improbably higher or lower than yours are, or would be.

Only realism combines safety with rewards. Optimism exposes you to needless risk, and pessimism leads to missed opportunities.

Finding the Income Ceiling in Your Present Practice

Once all doctors are working to capacity, practice income growth will usually be seriously slowed. Try to predict when that will occur, unless your practice is already there, at its *real* capacity. Also, as part of planning for the future, try to determine what your clinical capacity in patients served per day is or will be in your present operation.

Before planning an expansion project, remember that it won't be needed if a significantly higher *clinical* capacity in your existing office is feasible, which would happen if:

- The doctor(s) choose to work more hours per day, or more days per year
- The doctor(s) can give the needed care to more patients per day

But there will finally be a ceiling.

On the *dispensing* side income increases when more clinical patients:

- Stay for it
- Choose superior eyewear and lenses
- Choose multiple eyewear, sunglasses, etc.

The capacity needed in dispensing will be determined by the capacity of clinical services. Within limits, the present dispensing capacity can often be increased by reorganization and efficiencies in the eyewear and delivery operations. Effective steps can also be taken to increase the present capacity of your contact lens operation, vision therapy, sports vision, etc., but all will have an eventual ceiling.

When arrival at capacity slows or halts income growth, you will usually initiate your search for immediate and long-term answers. By seeing your need well in advance, you get an early start on the time-consuming process of planning immediate and long-term responses.

Capsule Summary: Causes of Growth in Patient Numbers after the Change, and How to Increase the Capacity of Your New Facility

After the change, clinical patient numbers will grow faster as a result of:

- Your announcements
- Referrals from patients enthusiastic about your new operation
- Your new marketing strategies
- The reaction of nonpatients to their positive perceptions of your office

Increased capacity to serve more clinical patients in your new facility will come from:

- More doctors
- More and better-trained staff
- More exam rooms per doctor
- Better efficiency and patient flow
- Better diagnostic techniques and instrumentation
- Computer applications, etc.

On the treatment side (dispensing eyewear, contact lenses, etc.), patient numbers will grow as signature fashion eyewear, superior performance lenses, and other innovations impress, attract, and interest patients. Higher treatment numbers will be accommodated by:

- More effective presentation of eyewear, lenses, and other needed items
- More and better-trained staff
- Better, more efficient techniques in all treatment procedures, etc.

Calculating Practice Capacity

With routine care appointments every twenty minutes for six hours with one hour for other "shorter time" services such as rechecks at ten minutes each, you will be able to serve 18 routine care patients per day, plus 6 more, for a total of 24 (18 plus 6), leaving the eighth hour for other things. With two doctors working on this basis, practice capacity is 48 a day.

If fifteen minutes is enough for routine care, two-doctor practice capacity per eight-hour day can be calculated by multiplying 24 routine patients (360 minutes [six hours] divided by fifteen minutes) plus 6 recheck patients, times two doctors, for a capacity of 60. You need to calculate how much growth can be handled before your practice again reaches capacity. This may reveal that you need space now for another doctor in the new facility later.

Net Income Clue That Your Space Is Now Too Small

Reduced *net* income with static or only slightly increased gross is another indication of "topped-up" space. As patient numbers reach practice capacity, you and your staff probably react by hiring staff to handle bottlenecks, but those extra people may not be kept busy enough. Steps to expand capacity taken without careful thought usually increase overhead faster than income, causing net income to drop, despite a slight improvement in gross.

Income Forecast: Who Should Do It?

To forecast additional annual income in your new facility, decide how it will be done, and then who will do it. Let's look first at who will do it.

You, guided by an ophthalmic management and marketing consultant (OMMC) with a strong track record with your profession, and perhaps your accountant, are the prime candidates. Because you are the one most familiar with the professional and administrative sides of your practice, *your contribution is vital*. You and an appropriate management consultant will also tend to know a lot about changes coming that will affect your profession, nationally, in your state, and in your community. You (with your OMMC's help and that of experienced colleagues) are thus best suited to forecast patient number growth for the first five years in your new facility.

Your accountant should translate your forecasted patient numbers growth into gross and net income growth. Your accountant may also, through familiarity with your eye-care practice and others, understand enough about your objectives, your preferred mode of practice, and your profession to participate effectively in practice management and major project planning.

Either way, as discussed in detail earlier, you should probably have the assistance of a reputable OMMC suitably experienced in your profession and your kind of practice. Get references from colleagues so you can make the most informed choice of the OMMC likely to be best for you.

When to Do Income Forecast

Do your first forecast early in planning, because it is an essential part of your project's feasibility study on which many action decisions will be based. After designing, just before you commit to construction, review and refine both the income forecast and the feasibility study, to verify your decisions.

Choosing the Income Forecast Method

Get the complete story of how your consultants plan to do this forecast, what it will cost, and whether it sounds sensible to you. You might discuss with your consultants whether a "good guidance" level of forecast is acceptable, rather than a more costly and time-consuming "extensive study."

Two Income Forecast Example Scenarios Needed

To forecast practice income, two key numbers are needed: average billing per patient, and number of patients served per year.

The necessary calculations are presented in two examples using assumed numbers (not from an existing practice—a legal point). Those numbers represent higher and lower scenarios of realities that have been achieved, and are used here in the hope that one will be close to your comfort level.

Two example calculations are needed because the assumed numbers must be close enough to your real numbers to make sense to you. "Average patient billing" and "number of patients served" occur at the higher and lower ends of the range too often among eye doctors for a single example based on the middle numbers to be credible with many readers. Too many might reject the process as not applicable to them.

This method simplifies a potentially complicated process by using familiar practice numbers and a process chosen for reasonable understanding by the nonaccountants among you. An alternative would be to use explanations instead of example numbers, but these would tend to be complex and difficult to understand (think of your income tax guide).

The first example calculation is titled "Average," for eye doctors who prefer working with numbers closer to the averages in statistically supported surveys of "average optometric patient billing" and "number of patients served." The second is "Higher Expectations," for those who expect to have a much bigger practice despite the doubts imposed by general survey statistics.

These scenarios are parallel in the sequence and details of their assumed figures and analysis. Only the numbers differ.

The numbers and calculations used have been reviewed by a respected authority in optometric statistics. Despite that, the experience of some optometrists will still suggest to them that one or both of these examples lack credibility. Also, these numbers will change over the years after this book is published.

The Income Forecast Calculation Process

1. *Find the present average billing per patient.* Divide last year's total income from patients by the total number of patients served in that year (regardless of the service each received).
2. *Find the average number of patients now being served per day.* Divide the total number of patients served in your previous year by the number of your "doctor-working days." Most optometrists serve their patients for 220 to 260 days per year (reported average of 245 in 1996).
3. *Forecast additional clinical patients in the first five years after your move.* Year one will have a big increase as your announcement cards act like recalls, and in response to other marketing. Year two growth may be slightly below year one. Year three might hold at the year two level, or increase a little. Growth speeds up again in year four. And, if capacity isn't reached in year four or early in five, the new growth rate could produce a fifth-year increase higher than year four. I am sometimes told that practice growth exceeded forecast (see Chapter 14). The best guide to this forecast of patient numbers will be the experience of colleagues.

"Average" Scenario

This doctor's practice may have already reached or be approaching its capacity. In this solo practice, appointments for routine eye care are every thirty minutes, a total of 14 patients during a fully booked seven-hour day (the eighth hour is for other things). In the new facility, routine appointments will need only twenty minutes (21 patients per seven-hour day), raising the capacity by 7 additional routine patients per day. "Additional" routine care patients per day will be those above the premove 14.

As shown in Figure 13-3, forecast the average number of additional patients that will be served per day during each of the practice's first five years in the new facility. In this case the fore-

Average Scenario
Forecast of Additional Patients Served Per Day After Move

Year After Move	Forecasted Each Year's Additional Clinical Patients Per day Per doctor	Forecasted TOTAL Additional Clinical Patients Per Day per Doctor In That year	Comments
Year 1	1.5	1.5	Strong first year growth
Year 2	1	2.5	Normal growth
Year 3	1	3.5	
Year 4	1.5	5	
Year 5	2	7	
		Total 19.5	

Figure 13–3 **Average scenario forecast of additional patients served per day after move. This shows that over the first five years in the new facility, the *average* number of additional clinical service patients per day would be approximately 4 (19.5 divided by 5). This number is only used for forecasting total additional annual income for the first five years, as described shortly.**

cast is based on the more moderate "average" scenario, closer to, but still five times higher than the 1996 survey averages for optometric practices in general.

Forecast New Average Billing Per Patient after Moving
In this example clinical patient billing should rise slowly. As previously noted, billing for treatment/dispensing should rise a little faster as patients choose better eyewear, superior performance lenses, etc. The total increase in average billing per patient is shown as significant but not large, as you will see from the assumed conservative numbers below.

1. *New average billing per patient, in new facility.*
   Average billing per patient before move: $143 (clinical fees
      $50, eyewear $93)
   Average billing per patient after move: $170 (clinical fees
      $57.50, eyewear $112.50)
   Percentage increase 19 percent
   Dollar increase $27.00

2. *Forecast of additional clinical income.*
   (a) From higher average fee for clinical services:
       Multiply $7.50 increase in average fees, times
       18 patients per day (previous 14, plus 4 new ones), times
       1 doctor (average over the 5 years), times
       245 "doctor" days per year, times
       5 years:
       Equals $165,375
   (b) From additional clinical patients:
       Multiply $50 previous average clinic fee, times
       4 more patients (5 year average per day—see chart), times
       1 doctor (the average for the 5 years), times
       245 "doctor" days per year, times
       5 years:
       Equals $245,000
   The total of (a) plus (b) is $410,375 forecasted additional clinical income for 5 years.

3. *Forecast of additional eyewear income.*
   (a) From increase in average eyewear billing per patient:
       Multiply $19.50 average billing increase per eyewear patient, times
       2,646 total average number of eyewear patients per year (60 percent of forecasted 4,410 clinical patients—11 per day for 245 days) times
       5 years:
       Equals $257,986
   (b) From additional eyewear patients:
       Multiply $93 previous average billing per eyewear patient, times
       880 additional eyewear patients per year (20 percent of 4,400, an increase to 80 percent from previous 60 percent of clinical patients), times
       5 years:
       Equals $409,200

The total of (a) plus (b) is $667,185 forecasted additional eyewear income for the 5 years. If that seems unrealistic to you, check with colleagues and/or change the numbers.

4. *Calculate total forecasted five-year additional gross income.*
   Add from above (as shown below):
   Additional clinical income of $419,562, plus
   Additional eyewear income of $667,185
   The total, $1,086,747, is the total forecasted five-year additional income.

5. *Managed care patients.*
   Subtract 20 percent from the $1,086,747, to get the lower
   final total of $869,398, because of less income from
   "managed care" patients. The 20 percent is arbitrary,
   as is explained near the end of the "Higher Expectations Scenario" that follows.

"Higher Expectations" Scenario

This possibly solo doctor sees routine care patients every twenty minutes (21 per seven-hour day). Practice capacity had been reached in the present office, so a second doctor must start with the move.

Over the first five years in the new facility the *average* number of additional clinical service patients per day would be 9 (45

Higher Expectations Scenario
Forecast of Additional Patients Served Per Day After Move

Year After Move	Forecased Each Year's Additional Clinical Patients Per Day Per Doctor	Forecasted TOTAL Additional Clinical Patients Per Day Per Doctor In That Year	Comments Second O.D. in practice from start.
Year 1	3	3	First year fastest growth
Year 2	2.5	5.5	First year momentum slowing
Year 3	3	8.5	Normal growth
Year 4	3.5	12	
Year 5	4	16	Doctors go to 15 minute appointments
		Total 45	

Figure 13–4   Higher expectations scenario forecast of additional patients served per day after move.

divided by 5). This number is only used for forecasting total additional annual income for the first five years, as described shortly.

Forecast New Average Billing Per Patient after Moving

Clinical patient billing in this example will rise faster because of fees for new procedures and higher fees for traditional ones. As previously noted, treatment/dispensing billing should rise more and faster as patients obtain new eyewear, multiple eyewear, sunglasses, etc., more often, and choose more costly eyewear or superior performance lenses. With a much stronger eyewear operation, this part of patient billing tends to yield the biggest increase in practice income. The following assumed figures represent a realistic forecast for some "higher-expectation" practices after the changes.

1. *New average billing per patient in new facility.*
   Average billing per patient before move: $185 (clinical fees $55, eyewear $130)
   Average billing per patient after move: $245 (clinical fees $65, Eyewear $180)
   Percentage increase: 32 percent
   Dollar increase: $60
   If that looks incorrect, check with colleagues who have made a particularly strong move including a powerful new eyewear operation, and/or change the numbers.

2. *Forecast of additional clinical income.*
   (a) From higher average fee for clinical services:
      Multiply $10 increase in average clinic fees, times
      30 patients per day, per doctor (previous 21, plus 9), times
      2 doctors, times
      250 doctor days per year, times
      5 years:
      Equals $750,000
   (b) From additional clinical patients:
      Multiply $55 pervious average clinic fee, times
      9 more patients (5 year average per day—see chart), times
      250 doctor days per year, times
      2 doctors, times

5 years:
Equals $1,237,500
The total of (a) plus (b) is, $1,987,500 forecasted additional five-year clinical income.

3. *Forecast of additional eyewear income.*
   (a) From increase in average eyewear billing per patient:
       Multiply $50 increase in average billing per eyewear
           patient, times
       6,000 total average number of eyewear patients per year
           (80 percent of forecasted 7,500 clinical patients—
           30 per day for 250 days) times
       5 years:
       Equals $1,500,000
   (b) From additional eyewear patients:
       Multiply $130 previous average billing per eyewear
           patient, times
       750 more eyewear patients per year (10 percent of
           7,500, up from previous 70 percent of clinical
           patients to 80 percent), times
       5 years:
   Equals $487,500
   The forecasted additional eyewear income for the five years,
   (a) plus (b) is $1,987,500.

4. *Calculate total forecasted five-year additional income.*
   Additional clinical income of $1,987,500, plus
   Additional eyewear income of $1,987,500
   The total, $3,975,000, is the forecasted five-year additional
   income.

In this practice, the $3,975,000 might be reduced 30 percent by the managed care income. This would drop the five-year additional income total to $2,782,500.

Impact of "Managed Care" (MC) on Income and Forecasts
Twenty percent was arbitrarily chosen as the reduction in practice income resulting from managed care (MC) in the "average" practice example forecast, and thirty percent in the "higher

FORECASTING WORKSHEET BEFORE AND AFTER THE PROJECT

REQUIRED INFORMATION FROM RECORDS
BEFORE PROJECT

1 Average Billing Per Patient Before Project   Clinical _____   Eyewear _____

2 Projected Average Billing Per Patient After The Project   Clinical _____   Eyewear _____

3 Average Number Of Patients Now Being Served Per Day (Before Project)   Clinical _____   Eyewear _____

PROJECTED ADDITIONAL PATIENTS

Forecasted Additional Clinical Patients Per Day Per Doctor	Forecasted Total Additional Clinical Patients Per Day Per Doctor
Year 1 _____	Year 1 _____
Year 2 _____	Year 2 _____
Year 3 _____	Year 3 _____
Year 4 _____	Year 4 _____
Year 5 _____	Year 5 _____
TOTAL _____	TOTAL _____

FORECAST ADDITIONAL INCOME
a) From Higher Average Fee For Clinical Services

MULTIPLY: ● Increase In Average Fees _____
x ● Forcasted New Total _____
x ● Number Of Doctors _____
x ● Number of Doctor's Days Per Year _____
x ● Over 5 Years _____
TOTAL _____   A) _____

b) From Additional Clinical Patients

MULTIPLY: ● Previous Average Clinical Fee _____
Average Number of Doctors For
x ● the 5 Years _____
x ● Number of "Doctor" Days Per Year _____
x ● 5 Years _____
TOTAL _____   B) _____

Add (a) Plus (b) For Forecasted Additional Income Per Year
TOTAL ADDITIONAL INCOME _____

FORECAST ADDITIONAL EYEWEAR INCOME
a) From Increase In Average Eyewear Billing Per Patient

MULTIPLY: ● Average Billing Increase Per Eyewear Patient _____
x ● Total Average Number Of Eyewear Patients Per Year _____
x ● 5 Years _____
TOTAL _____   A) _____

b) From Additional Eyeware Patients

MULTIPLY: ● Previous Average Eyewear Billing Per Eyewear Patient _____
x ● Forecasted Additional Eyewear Patients Per Year _____
x ● 5 Years _____
TOTAL _____   B) _____

Add (a) Plus (b) For Forecasted Additional Eyewear Income Per Year
TOTAL ADDITIONAL EYEWEAR INCOME _____

SUMMARY
For Total Forecasted 5 Year Gross Additional Income

ADD: Total Additional Clinical Income _____
Total Additional Eyewear Income _____

TOTAL GROSS ADDITIONAL 5 YEAR INCOME _____

Figure 13–5   Forecasting worksheet before and after the project.

expectation" forecast. Those percentages emphasize why MC income should be in the forecast. MC income's impact on proposed projects can range from zero with no MC patients, to critical (perhaps dictating a very different project, or none).

Watch your national association's survey reports of changes in practice income caused by average billing per MC patient and number of MC patients being served. Either include MC income as a part of your forecast of total income, or make a separate forecast of MC income, in the same way as presented above, for income from the "independent" side of the practice. Then factor the results into the picture.

Find Additional Net Income
Generated by Your Forecast of the Gross

Additional net income of the practice is the return on investment available to pay for your project and get additional practice income. Your accountant should calculate the approximate additional net income generated by your forecasted gross over the first five years in your new office.

Set Your Budget Limit

Ask your accountant and/or management consultant to calculate from your forecasted additional net income how much you can justify investing to get this increase in net income. The answer will be your budget limit. Your financing (borrowing) needs will be reduced by your personal investment.

CHAPTER 14

Colleague Questionnaire Report

A Reality Report

The "Questionnaire Report" that follows throws light on the experiences, results, and thoughts of eye doctors (optometrists only) who completed projects—their reality.

Colleague Calls and Visits:
Guarding the Time of Your Colleague

Throughout the book you have been urged, as you are again here, to contact colleagues who have "been there." Their unique experience-based knowledge can greatly help your project. Find out if they can take the time to talk to you. With some (see below), request permission to visit.

Colleagues who agree to your request will obviously be giving you the generous gifts of their time and data. Although many will be willing or happy to answer your questions and give you information, some may quite understandably decline. They may have already dealt with a number of such appeals, and perhaps had no similar assistance available when planning their own project. Also, as you would expect, the majority will tend to be very busy.

Beyond your normal considerate behavior, the foregoing are additional good reasons for you to use as little of each willing colleague's time as feasible, while recognizing that your interview call is likely to be relatively long even when you hold your questions to a minimum. Even when the goodwill is there, you should still diligently guard this generous person's time.

To help you and your colleague minimize this phone time, study the report that follows, which presents answers to a questionnaire sent to optometrists. It reports on completed projects of this kind. The answers there should make many of your possible questions unnecessary.

Plan these contacts with colleagues well, for their sake and yours. Include in your short list of questions only those that are most important to you and are not answered to your satisfaction in the questionnaire report. At the same time, although short, your list should be inclusive enough so repeat calls are unnecessary.

Try to call at least two or three of these colleagues (more would be better), so the information on which your project planning depends will be more extensive and thus more reliable.

Perhaps confine your first phone contact to a brief explanation of your request. Ask permission to send your list of questions and make a telephone appointment to discuss those questions at a time convenient to your colleague. As possible, make that phone appointment for a time of day when your colleague is relaxed and free from the usual office pressures (perhaps at home in the evening, after dinner).

If you are requesting a visit, remind your colleague that you will be delighted to be shown around by a staff member, so you won't be using much of your colleague's time. You might also ask for permission to take pictures, if she/he is comfortable with it.

The Range of Information You Can Get

Don't be put off by inconsistent reports. Choose which reports sound closest to your picture. Despite any differences, much of the reality revealed by them will be advice that is wide ranging, soundly based, and hard-to-get. Simply by hearing and seeing the results experienced by colleagues who took the action you are considering, you will be getting substantial benefit. This is your best way of checking the claims, reports, and ideas you are given by people who say they can guide you (myself included, as in this book).

As much as possible, try to find and then contact colleagues who practice in situations not too different from yours. Most designers and management consultants know the circumstances of their clients' practices and could direct you. Otherwise, try the "optical grapevine."

You will get stories on a range of experience topics. These should include:

- Return on investment
- Costs
- Referrals to evaluations of and sources of guidance/ assistance
- Size of facility you should be considering
- Time needed for planning, and then for all other steps to completion
- Methods of project control
- Problems against which to guard yourself
- A promising path for financing

Your Lists of Questions

Consider making two lists. The first will have questions to ask in your phone calls and visits. This relatively short list will have questions important to *you* that are unanswered in the report below.

Your second list, for your eyes only, should cover things for you to look at and think about during a visit.

If you are planning a startup office, your list will contain questions specific to startup. Obviously you would try to find a doctor who owns a "recent" (two or three years) startup practice. Although most of these questions would be on a "regular" list, the startup list will still differ.

Introduction to Questionnaire (Sent to Optometrists Only)

The questionnaire that follows was developed to collect information from optometrists who had completed new-office projects. It was intended to save the time of doctors who may be phoned or visited by colleagues who are considering or planning a project, by answering in advance many questions they would be asked, often repeatedly by different callers.

The questionnaire was sent to 111 optometrists who had completed new facility projects in the United States and Canada. Seventy-nine replies were received. The largely anonymous answers were statistically analyzed, edited, and then reported. The practice design and installation projects in the questionnaire are a specialized sample because all involved the work of Larry Funston, designer, and usually myself.

Although the questionnaire answers could satisfy your need on many topics, the answers should definitely *not* be viewed as a substitute for your phone calls, your visits to see some of the facilities and the practices they contain, or your contacts with designers and consultants in the fields involved.

Confidentiality

All who answered the questionnaire were assured of confidentiality. The answers were processed into computer printouts by a minimum number of people who had no known connection with the ophthalmic professions or industry, and no known stake in the answers.

Writing the Questions and Processing the Answers

I wrote questions that I felt needed to be investigated, and had help from a professional experienced in questionnaires, so the questions would be phrased to produce answers suitable for useful analysis.

All of the answers received were typed into a single document that was then given to an independent professional in this field of "questionnaire and answer" information processing. He is a friend and university professor in these subjects and is very active as a consultant. He reports that the sample size (seventy-nine completed questionnaires received) permits information that is potentially useful, but not authoritative. He used a small group of his postgraduate students to input the data and analyze it using suitable software.

The result was more than 100 pages of printout analysis. The consultant, with a little help from me, interpreted those pages into the report that follows.

Some questions requested a descriptive answer, resulting in long lists of different replies. All but one of these lists have been grouped into categories, as indicated in the report. In the one exception (Question 31—"What would you do differently, if you were starting a project now?"), categorization seemed impossible, so the entire list of answers is in the report.

It seemed desirable to separate and report individually on the replies from optometrists practicing in Canada and the United States. Although optometry in the two countries has much in common (as observable in the report), some of the differences produce entirely different answers—for example, the different meanings of the term "managed care."

The Structure of the Report

The answers to each question are presented separately, in sequence. The following points are addressed:

- Why the question was asked
- The answers from the United States and Canada shown separately, but side by side
- Any comments that seem appropriate
- At the end of each question, the point(s) I felt have "Possible significance"

Report on Questionnaire Answers

(Percentages represent how often this answer occurred, as a percentage of the total answers.)

1. This question has two parts.
   a. Why did you decide to take on your project?
   b. What were your prime objectives?

   Reason for questions: Learn why optometrists wanted to tackle such a big project
   Replies: (Percentages of replies per answer)

	United States	Canada
a. Appearance and image	24.7%	23.1%
b. Space	24.7	21.1
c. Efficiency and flow	13.7	24.3
d. Growth	12.6	7.6
e. Revenue	7.7	6.7
f. Quality of care and modernization	5.6	6.5
g. Comfort	3.3	5.6
h. Competition	3.3	0
i. Location and parking	2.7	0
j. Cost	0	2.9

Possible significance: The priority given to each of the objectives suggests that doctor interest was mainly in the means of achieving her/his version of success, rather than on the success itself. The low priority of "competition" is of interest.

2. **Would you now say that these goals were achieved?**

   Reason for question: Get a measure of project results per objectives.

   Possible significance: This supports having an impressive, outstanding office.

Yes	91.7%	100%

3. **How many years have you been in this office?**

   Reason for question: So reader can judge the perspective behind the answers.

   Possible significance: Perhaps a surprising percentage of doctors reporting have had six years or more to observe and consider the results they reported.

One to two years	0%	8.0%
Three to five years	23.9	14.0
Six to ten years	28.6	32.0
Eleven to fifteen years	42.9	34.0
Sixteen and over years	4.8	12.0

4. **What are the data on your market area?**

   Reason for question: Permit reader to judge if some of the markets that were reported relate to his/hers.

   a. **Market Population at New Office**

Up to 23,000	28.6%	27.5%
25,000 to 49,000	28.5	25.4
50,000 to 90,000	14.3	13.7
100,000 to 400,000	28.6	29.4
1 to 3 million	0	4

   b. **Competition:** In both countries, a wide variety and amount of competition was reported, both in specific and general terms, but no grouping seemed to emerge that would provide useful information.

   c. **Economy in Market**

   Possible significance: The few projects that are in larger cities (over 400,000) is notable, and the not surprising choice of doctors to proceed where their local economy is "good to excellent."

Weak and depressed	8.4%	11.2%
Fair	4.2	11.1
Good + medium + stable	66.7	59.4
Strong + excellent	8.3	9.3
No answer	12.5	9.3

5. What are your patient demographics?

Reason for question: Permit reader to judge if some of these practices resemble his/hers.

a. Patient Age

Seniors	24.0%	23.6%
Middle age	17.6	25.6
Young adult	20.1	18.4
Children	17.6	11.3
No answer	20.8	20.4

b. Patient income (Note: $1.00 Can. = approx. $.66 U.S.)
(I expected that these would be approximate levels based on local information, sometimes reported in the local press.)

U.S	Canada (approx. equivalent to U.S. figures on left.)		
$12,500	$20,000	0%	5.6%
$18,600	$30,000	33.3	16.7
$19,000 to 25,000	$31,000 to 40,000	33.3	16.7
$31,000 to 43,000	$50,000 to 70,000	33.3	55.6
$67,000	$100,000	0	5.6

c. Employment picture

Weak	6.3%	6.6%
Average + good	43.8	63.1
Excellent	16.8	8.6
Unsure + variable	4.2	3.2
No answer	29.2	18.5

Possible significance: Since this picture seems to show reasonably balanced patient demographics, the conditions involved should apply to a wide range of those considering a project.

6. **In pre-design planning of your project, did you work with optometric management/marketing consultants?**

   Reason for question: Did project-minded optometrists value this third-party advice?

Yes	62.5%	50.0%
No	33.3	48.1
No answer	4.2	1.9

   Possible significance: A sizable number of optometrists sought guidance from this professional source, suggesting confidence.

7. **How would you rate what they did for you in that planning? (Among those using service)**

   Reason for question: Give readers a report on project O.D. satisfaction with this service. Ratings were on a scale from 1, No Help, to 10, Extremely Helpful that are reduced to 5 categories below.

No help	5.6%	10.3%
Helpful + Truly Helpful	22.2	27.6
Very Helpful	16.7	20.7
Extremely Helpful	22.2	13.8
Indispensable + Essential	16.7	27.6

   Possible significance: Those who obtained guidance from these consultants were almost always pleased with the result.

8. **What was the role of your accountant?**

   Reason for question: Did "Project O.D.'s" tend to seek advice from their accountants?

Not involved	33.3%	37.0%
Somewhat involved	37.5	51.9
Involved	20.8	9.5
Very involved	4.2	1.9
Ultimate authority	4.2	0

   Possible significance: These optometrists seemed disinclined to seek project guidance from their accountants. This could be of interest to accountants, who are often involved in management planning in other fields.

9. **How many doctors are there in your practice? (After the project)**

   Reason for question: Guide readers on planning for growth and financial planning. (Error in question: Should have asked how many *more* doctors after the project.)

   a. **Full time doctors now in the practice**

One	54.5%	46.1%
Two	27.3	26.9
Three	4.5	15.4
Four and over	13.6	11.5

   b. **Part time doctors now in the practice**

None	47.4%	38.9%
One	42.1	41.7
Two	10.5	11.1
More than two	0	8.4

Possible significance: Growth in the number of doctors would indicate considerable practice growth after the project, for which adequate space must be planned. And income growth forecasted from additional doctors would have to be factored into budgeting.

10. **Since moving did you, or will you soon have another doctor?**

    Reason for question: Guidance on growth planning.

No	37.5%	42.6%
Unsure	20.8	13.0
Yes	41.7	44.4

Possible significance: The same as the preceding.

11. **How much "doctor time" do you schedule for:**
    a. Full exam
    b. Re-check
    c. Contact lens check

    Reason for question: Data for analyzing the practice's patient care capacity in the new facility, which will control what income maximum and return-on-investment is possible.

    a. Time for a full exam

Ten minutes	0%	3.8%
Fifteen minutes	16.7	3.8
Twenty minutes	16.7	42.3
Twenty-five minutes	4.2	7.7
Thirty minutes	50.0	40.7
Forty or forty-five minutes	12.5	1.9

b. Time for a re-check

Five minutes	9.5%	0%
Ten minutes	38.1	33.3
Fifteen minutes	52.4	49.1
Twenty minutes and over	0	17.7

c. Time for a contact lens check

Five minutes	8.7%	5.9%
Ten and eight minutes	43.4	31.4
Fifteen minutes	47.8	47.1
Twenty minutes and over	0	15.8

Possible significance: The need for both care excellence and practice income will dictate careful targeting of, and designing for practice capacity. The above data may help optometrists base space need on time with patient.

12. **How many days per year (estimation) is there a doctor serving patients?**
    (The data here are similar to that in the recently released Workforce Study of the AOA, presented in the *AOA News*.)

    Reason for question: Another key factor in finding the practice capacity in new facility.

Less than 200 days	4.5%	8.4%
200 to 220 days	18.2	29.2
221 to 250 days	36.4	39.4
251 to 270 days	9.1	6.3
271 to 325 days	31.7	16.7

Possible significance: The opposing pulls of income need versus all the valid reasons for doctor's absence affects days worked, and thus practice capacity. It is of interest that the

"271 to 325 day category" above shows an unexpectedly high preference among these postproject optometrists.

13. **How do you now do a preexam?**
    a. **Yourself**
    b. **Optometric assistant**
    c. **What instruments do you use?**
    d. **Is there a bottleneck?**
    e. **How would you like to change it?**
    (The report will omit "c," which resulted in a list so varied that it provides little guidance.)

    Reason for the questions: Help in design planning for the changing preexam function.

    a. Yourself (the doctor does the preexam)

Always	12.5%	14.9%
Never	62.5	53.7
Sometimes + Rarely	16.7	27.8
No answer	8.3	3.7

    b. Optometric assistant

Almost always + usually	12.5%	11.2%
Always	70.8	59.3
Never	12.5	9.3
Sometimes	0	13.0
No answer	4.2	7.4

    d. Is there a bottleneck?

No	62.4%	48.1%
Yes + Occasionally	33.4	40.8
No answer	4.2	11.1

e. How would you like to change it?

Improve capacity through assistants	8.4%	14.8%
Improve capacity through equipment	21.0	5.7
Improve capacity through more space	12.6	13.1
Improve capacity by adjusting appointment times	0	3.8
Doctors increase their pretest capacity	0	3.8
No Changes Needed + Unsure	8.4	11.1
No answer	49.6	48.1

Possible significance: The percentage of optometrists reporting a bottleneck here is smaller than I expected from conversations with postproject optometrists, but its size still suggests that design planning involve a thorough study of the forecasted capacity needed, and the best strategy for getting that capacity.

14. Are your patient records computerized?
    a. Full patient record?
    b. Financial records only?
    c. Do you have a paper backup?
    d. Do you have electronic backup?
    e. How does your staff rate it?
    f. What is the name of the computer program you use?
    (The report omits "f," a list too varied to be helpful here.)

Reason for the question: Guidance and emphasis on design planning to meet this need.

a. Full patient record computerized?

No	66.7%	70.4%
Yes	20.8	27.8
Partial + Some	8.4	0
No answer	4.2	1.9

b. Financial records only computerized?

No	20.8%	24.1%
Yes	66.7	57.4
No answer	12.5	18.5

c. Do you have a paper backup?

No	25.0%	38.9%
Yes	62.5	46.3
No answer	12.5	14.9

d. Do you have electronic backup?

No	4.2%	11.1%
Yes	83.3	79.6
No answer	12.5	9.3

e. How does your staff rate it? (1, No Help, to 10, Extremely Helpful)

Five and Below	22.6%	8.9%
Six and above	77.4	91.1

Possible significance: This supports the established point that fully computerized records are becoming standard, and thus should be included in design planning.

15. **Does your practice offer the services of a "visiting" ophthalmologist?**

    Reason for the question: O.D. guidance in predesign planning.

No	62.5%	81.5%
Yes	37.5	13.0
No answer	0	5.5

    a. **If yes, what spaces are used by this M.D.?**
    b. **Any comments?**

    The answers to these questions are omitted, as providing insufficient useful information.

    Possible significance: Since this question doesn't reveal the key matter of rate of acceptance of this new mode of practice, it provides little guidance in an important area of design planning.

16. **If you feel comfortable about reporting it,**
    a. **What is your average (median) billing per patient?**
    b. **How much has it changed since your project?**

    Reason for these questions: Guidance for financial planning, budget limit, etc. (Answers came from 62.5% of the U.S. optometrists who answered the questionnaire, and 50% of the Canadians.)

    a. **What is your median billing per patient? ($U.S. and $Canadian are reported)**

Less than $100	6.7%	25.2%
$100 to $149	13.4	18.0
$150 to $199	6.7	21.5

$200 to $249	40.0	25.1
$250 to $299	13.4	0.8
$300 to $325	19.8	0

b. How much has it changed since your project? (Increased)

Zero	0%	9.5%
Up to $14	8.3	33.3
$15 to 29	33.4	38.0
$30 to $44	16.7	9.5
$45 to $99	24.8	9.5
$100 and over	16.7	0

Possible significance: This is essential to the calculation of anticipated income in the new facility, which directly affects the budget limit. Fee levels certainly look better in the United States.

17. **Managed Care**
    a. **What approximate percentage of your practice is "managed care?"**
    b. **How much has it changed since your project?**

    Reason for question: Guidance on impact of managed care on income and facility investment.

    ("Managed care" isn't the same thing in Canada, so this report is for the United States only.)

    a. **What approximate percentage of your practice is "managed care?"**

5% to less than 30%	26.7% of reporting group
30% to less than 60%	43.4
60% to less than 90%	30.4

b. **How much has it changed since your project? (Income change *expected*)**

0 to 24% income reduction expected	77.7% of reporting group
25% to 49%	5.6
50% to 74%	0
75% to 95%	16.7

Possible significance: Obviously, this also is a critical factor in calculating expected income in the new facility, which directly affects project budget limit. Check for trend information in "managed care" in your professional journals.

18. **How much is "managed care" affecting your income? (This is a continuation of the previous question.)**

19. **In the first five years after the change, was/is patient numbers growth as forecasted?**

    Reason for question: How reliable were the planning forecasts of practice growth?

As forecast	8.3%	3.8%
Above forecast	58.4	46.3
Below forecast	12.5	24.1
No answer	20.8	26.7

Possible significance: This indicates that forecasting of practice growth after the project is seriously low, which would unnecessarily and perhaps harmfully hold down the forecasted level of income, and thus the project budget limit.

20. **How long did or will it take, to pay off your project (do not include real estate costs)?**

    Reason for the question: Did this project produce an appropriate return-on-investment?

Five years or less	40.0%	63.2%
Six to ten years	30.0	28.5
Eleven to twenty years	30.0	8.1

Possible significance: This should provide guidance in setting a realistic, but "not too soft" target of time for your investment to be paid off while yielding an adequate return-on-investment.

21. **Has your return-on-investment been**

(Ranked from 1, Very dismal, to 10, Just super!) Again, the ten categories were condensed to five. Reason for question: Evidence of the effectiveness of the investment.

Poor	8.6%	0 %
Fair	0	6.1
Good	39.1	22.4
Excellent	30.4	48.9
Super	21.7	22.4

Possible significance: As in the preceding question, this provides guidance for financial planning, and design planning for return-on-investment. The report suggests that forecasting may have been low fairly often, and thus could have held back the investment, possibly resulting in a less effective project.

22. **Rank where most of the increased income came from:**
    a. **Additional patients served?**
    b. **Increased return per patient?**
    c. **The clinical side of the practice?**
    d. **The dispensing side?**

Reason for the question: Guidance in budget forecasting and design planning.

a. Additional patients served	61.1%	51.0%
b. Increased return per patient	38.9	42.9
No answer	0	6.1
c. The clinical side of the practice	35.3%	33.3%
d. The dispensing side	50.0	57.2
e. Operating costs reduced (See question 23)	14.7	9.4

Possible significance: The "additional patients served" figure emphasizes the need to design adequate, balanced patient care capacity for the foreseeable future, and the "increased return per patient" figure indicates the need for a design that supports those functions that yield the increased return.

23. **Were operating costs per patient reduced?**
    a. Is it notable extra income?

    Reason for question: Guidance in budget forecasting and design planning.

    a. Is it notable income? (See question 22e above.)

    Possible significance: Clearly this is the least productive source of additional income after the project, but it can be significant. It should be addressed in design and operational planning.

24. **Do you think that perceptions of your new office helped much in speeding up practice growth? (1, Negative, to 10, Positive) This report was reduced to four categories.**

    Reason for question: Guidance on importance of public/patient perceptions of facility.

Not significantly	4.3%	0 %
Significantly	21.7	3.8
Strongly	39.1	37.7
Very strongly	47.8	58.5

Possible significance: This draws attention to and emphasizes the contribution to practice building and thus the success of this kind of venture of patient and public perceptions of you and your practice.

25. **Rank in what ways the appearance of your office strengthened your practice:**
    a. Income
    b. The confidence of patients
    c. The respect of other health care professionals
    d. Other ways—please list and rank

    Reason for these questions: Guidance in perceptions planning.

Income	4.8%	21.7%
Confidence of patients	85.8	68.3
Respect of other health care professionals	4.8	8.3
Other	4.8	1.7

Possible significance: Although the contribution to "income" receives scant support, "patient confidence" (which was very strong) directly affects practice income. The choice of "patient confidence" by so many optometrists in the report suggests that this is the dominant way in which this economic benefit is delivered by the new facility.

26. **Have patient referrals in response to your eyewear room generated an important number of new clinical patients?**

    Reason for question: Does eyewear operation contribute significantly to clinical growth?

Yes	54.2%	72.2%
Unsure	16.7	27.8
No	29.2	0

Possible significance: This supports the expected benefit to the practice of a uniformly high, impressive level of performance and appearance in the eyewear operation.

27. **Do you have computer terminals in your eyewear room?**
    a. How helpful is it? (1, Not helpful, to 10, Extremely helpful) Answers are condensed to four categories.

Reason for question: Guidance in design planning for computer terminals in eyewear.

No	54.2%	51.9%
Yes	37.5	44.4
No answer	8.3	3.7

a. How helpful is it?

Not helpful	12.5%	0 %
Fairly helpful	0	12.0
Very helpful	50.0	32.0
Extremely helpful	37.5	56.0

Possible significance: The support for this computer application indicates that it should be planned carefully for its operation in the eyewear area design.

28. **Do, or did you have a problem of too much heat from display lighting in eyewear room?**

Reason for question: Important point, discussed in the text.

Yes	58.3%	64.9%
No	41.7	35.1

Possible significance: This emphasizes the need for a much better understanding of display lighting and air conditioning. See Chapter 7, "Eyewear Area Design Criteria."

29. **How do you present today's superior performance lenses and new lens options?**

    Reason for the question: Identify whether there is an unfilled need (opportunity) here.

Samples	41.7%	36.8%
Verbal (doctor and/or staff)	38.3	10.2
Don't do it	0	36.3
No answer	20.0	16.6

    Possible significance: This question and the answers don't help identify a need for better techniques here. (Its importance to patient benefit and practice income should still indicate a need for creative design planning.)

30. **Do you wish you had taken more space?**
    a. If so, how much more?

    Reason for the question: Guidance on conflict between space need and cost.

Yes	41.7%	46.3%
No	50.0	42.6
Unsure	4.2	9.3
No answer	4.2	1.9

    a. How much more space?

100 through 300 sq. ft.	30.0%	15.0%
500 through 600 sq. ft.	40.0	30.0
800 through 1,000 sq. ft.	20.0	30.0
1,500 through 2,000 sq. ft.	0	20.0
4,000 through 5,000 sq. ft.	10.0	5.0

Possible significance: report emphasizes again that space is a critical planning decision, with strong support for planning it very carefully.

31. **What would you do differently, if you were starting a project now?**

    Reason for question: Identify items that should probably not be overlooked in planning.
    United States

- Have an area for sunwear.
- Carefully examine plans, especially desk space and storage. Use local contractor for an on-site supervisor.
- Design a smaller office to reduce overhead. HMOs don't pay more if you have a bigger overhead.
- Eliminate the waiting room. Add one more refracting lane?
- Get more space.
- Give more space to the eyewear selecting area.
- Given what I had to work with—nothing.
- I wish I'd (1) known how much this would help, (2) had more to purchase more space.
- I would make the front desk more private.
- Increase CL and optical lab size. Better storage for records, decorations, financial data, etc.
- Increase space for office staff, administration.
- More file space, larger pre-test, V.T. room, more elaborate frame selection area.
- More open concept so patient feels more comfortable browsing while waiting—and also so we'd use less staff.
- More storage.
- More storage spaces, bigger CL lab and optical lab.
- Not much other than size, and better lighting on frames as well as patients seeing themselves.
- Not spend so much money or go so high class—patients don't care and it made us broke.
- Nothing.
- Put eyewear room at front of office. Make CL storage room bigger and CL training room smaller. Put cleaning supply area on first floor.

- Scale down the larger office.
- Storage, maybe 1,000 to 1,500 sq. ft. in basement.
- Try to line up the money first.
- Will need more exam lanes and work-up area for third party as it grows.

CANADA

- 1. Prefer to buy a building. 2. Have two stories. 3. Space for computerizing. 4. More area for computerizing.
- 1. More space for business office/reception area. 2. Provide space for computers, which was not considered fifteen years ago.
- Begin five years sooner.
- Better costing estimations, more quotes, better contract.
- Better lighting in dispensary for patients picking up their new glasses.
- Bigger, more independent access to each department—clinical, CL, dispensary.
- Buy a building.
- Change flow. More sunglass display. More pretest space.
- Compare more design consultants.
- Design more space for work areas and labs.
- Get ready for new millennium and even faster eye care.
- Ground floor location.
- Find a way to downsize without losing critical areas.
- Have more space if possible.
- Have frame room visible from waiting room. Do not separate reception and accounts payable as both areas could be better covered for patients if one staff member was away from her area. Waiting room and desks should be seen by all front line staff.
- I would actually go smaller in general, have smaller frame inventory, etc. My facility has worked out very well. Some people estimate that it's two years old when it's actually ten. Ten years ago I was quite naive about business matters.
- I would make more space for computers as none in office when I started.

- Larger area.
- Larger frame adjustment area.
- Larger frame and waiting room, and more storage. This is now needed because of extra doctors—all was OK for many years. The question is how far ahead should you plan your space requirements? Should you move or expand every ten years? Space costs money.
- Larger preexam and Rx delivery.
- Look at space for an extra pretest area.
- Make street side better. Change dispensary. Wire for VDT.
- More carefully watch construction costs.
- More space. Larger dispensing area. A little more attention to patient flow.
- More space.
- More space and everything first class. Skylights? (or better ones). More storage.
- Not much.
- Nothing
- Not much—I would arrange my exam room a bit differently, but that is because of technique changes.
- Not much.
- Not much—Do a better job with lighting.
- Not much!
- Nothing
- Plan for more growth than you anticipate.
- Spend less. This relates to frozen or reduced health care fees.
- Stay on one floor.
- Take slightly more space.
- We have been unhappy with the carpet recommended.
- Wider space. Three exam rooms.

Possible significance: Readers with a strong interest in statistical analysis will without doubt find ways of recognizing trends in the foregoing list. I encourage this, but backed away for two reasons: (a) I wanted the entire list shown so readers would be able to see the whole picture, and correctly perceive that nothing had been omitted. (b) I am uneasy about categorizing many of the answers, although the basis for some groupings is easily spotted.

Despite the above, this report suggests that the optometrists involved found their project to be a learning experience. Even with professional advice from one or more sources, some feel that with today's knowledge they would do quite a few important things differently. As you read their comments, you may pick up ideas that you recognize as valuable.

32 and 33 combined

32. How many people did you previously employ?
(It was assumed that this would exclude doctors)

33. How many do you now employ (excluding doctors)

Reason for the questions: 32, indication of practice size at time decision made to invest; 33, indication of practice growth after the project.

	United States		Canada	
	Before	After	Before	After
One employee	18.2%	0%	10.6%	3.9%
Two	0	0	34.0	11.8
Three	18.2	4.3	19.1	15.7
Four	27.3	21.7	6.4	13.8
Five	18.2	13.0	6.4	9.8
Six	4.5	13.0	6.4	5.9
Seven	0	0	4.3	7.8
Eight	13.6	0	6.4	5.9
Nine	0	4.3	0	2.0
Ten	0	13.0	0	9.8
Eleven	0	8.7	0	0
Twelve	0	4.3	2.1	2.0
Fourteen and over	0	17.7	4.2	11.9

Possible significance: Despite the different experience in the United States and Canada, this is further data on practice growth after the project. Most optometrists will be comfortable accepting "number of employees" as a loose but useful measure of practice size.

About You

Reasons for questions: years in practice, age of the doctor at approximate time of project, number of projects that were repeats, and present size of practice in terms of patients served per year, should help the doctor/reader learn whether the circumstances resemble his/hers.

34. **Year graduated from Optometry**

Before 1964	0 %	4.0%
1964 through 1970	12.9	12.0
1971 through 1975	12.9	14.0
1976 through 1980	43.3	36.0
1981 through 1985	21.7	14.0
1986 through 1990	0	6.0
1991 through 1994	4.3	4.0

35. **Year opened in this location**

Before 1970	4.2%	3.9%
1971 through 1975	4.2	4.0
1976 through 1980	8.4	9.8
1981 through 1985	8.4	15.7
1986 through 1990	33.3	35.3
1991 through 1995	33.3	20.6
1996 through 1998	8.3	9.9

36. Number of previous locations

None (This is my startup location)	13.6%	14.0%
One previous location	50.0	60.0
Two	22.7	20.0
Three	9.2	6.0
Four	4.5	0

37. Year you were born

1940 and earlier	4.3%	4.0%
1941 through 1945	17.4	8.0
1946 through 1950	13.0	18.4
1951 through 1955	56.7	30.7
1956 through 1960	4.3	30.8
1961 through 1965	4.3	6.1
1969	0	2.0

Possible significance of answers to questions 34 through 37: Optometrists thinking about a possible project often want to know if it seems sensible at their age, stage in their career, at this time, etc. By seeing the personal data on their colleagues who made the move, they can get guidance in making their decision.

38. **Size of practice measured in number of patients served per year:** (It was assumed that this would include patient visits for any paid service.)

Zero through 3,000 patients per year	0 %	14.0%
3,001 through 6,000	45.8	33.3
6,001 through 9,000	29.2	17.5
9,001 through 12,000	8.3	15.6
12,001 through 15,000	8.3	6.6

Over 15,000	4.2	3.7
No answer	4.2	9.3

Possible significance: This seems quite puzzling. Practice growth in patient numbers is not as high as I expected from the earlier answer to the question on sources of practice growth that identified increased patient numbers as the leader.

Comments on the Report

Readers are encouraged to draw conclusions from this report, particularly as a subject pertains to their circumstances and interests.

It seems evident to me, that this report offers at least the following benefits:

- A limited "checklist" of topics and their components that could merit exploration by an eye doctor considering a new office project
- Partial answers to some critical questions, particularly in and after judging whether the guidance information pertains to the circumstances of your practice
- An appreciation of the individuality and range of differences in doctors and circumstances that indicate the need for *your* picture to be investigated thoroughly, and then responded to specifically in all project planning

In Closing

Your information gathering should by now have reached its target, permitting you to know whether and why you are comfortable with your proposed venture and to make your project decisions with confidence

Now, as an old (Newfoundland?) saying goes, "May ye have the wind at yer back with a downhill pull."

Index

Cost(s)
   building shell, 318
   choosing a location and, 46
   common, 316–317
   cutting, 319
   design and, 269–270, 271–272
   estimating, 316–320
   expanding present office and,
      56–57
   exterior contractor costs, 317
   feasibility, 315–320
   foundation, 318
   guesstimating, 319–320
   interior contractor costs,
      316–317
   lot development, 318
   related to benefit for functions,
      77–78
   unexpected, 318–319

D
Decision making, 1
   for existing practice, 3
Deficiency list, 290–292
Delivery station for new and
      replacement contact lenses,
      122–123
Demographics of patients, 350
Design criteria
   clinical functions, 75–114
   contact lens service, 115–125
   definition, 19
   examples of, 19
   eyewear area, 127–199
   eyewear delivery services and
      lens production lab,
      213–237
   lens application functions,
      201–211
   objectives, 17–28
   objectives versus, 19–20
Design process, 264–266
   approval, 272
   conceptual, 268–273

flow chart, 295–297
other doctors' designs, using,
   273–274
renderings, 272–273
steps in, 269–273
Designer-consultant, expectations
   from, 255–297
   advice on project choices you
      make, 262–263
   compromise in planning, 263
   conceptual design process,
      268–273
   considering consultants,
      255–256
   contractor and designer in one
      operation, 308–310
   duplication of contractor serv-
      ices, 313
   individualized to you, 292–294
   location choice, 258
   ongoing connection, 295
   predesign planning team, 255
   problems to be solved and your
      other objectives, 266–268
   process and responsibilities of
      designer up to conceptual
      design, 264–266
   process flow chart, 295–297
   project feasibility, 256
   project management, 281–292
   qualifications, 263
   renderings, 272–273
   role of you and your designer,
      293–294
   size of space needed, 257–258
   subjects for advice, 256–260
   timing, 258–260
   using other doctors' designs,
      273–274
   views of doctor/owner and,
      266–267
   why work with, 260–262
   working drawings alternative,
      281

Sunglasses and other product presentation displays, 228–229
Superiority, patient recognition of, 135
Supplies station and display, contact lens services, 123
Surgery to avoid wearing glasses, 131–132
Surgery room, minor, 102
Surgical center room, ambulatory, 102

T
Targeting your patients and eyewear, 133–135
Taste and perceptions, 40–42
Tax benefit of owning location, 70
Tax picture and owning location, 73
Technician/assistant work stations and their location, 93–95
Telephone placement to avoid voice mail, 82–83
Testing room, special, 102
Time spent with patients, 21, 353–355
Timing in life of your practice and location, 48–49
Traffic passing, 44, 45, 67
Training area, contact lens, 121–122
Try-on station and lighting, 186

V
Venture analysis, 315–316
Videotapes for patients, 87, 92–93
on contact lens, 119, 120
for eyewear selection, 194–195

at inner waiting for eyewear delivery, 224–226
on lens, 208
on repair parts availability, 224
room for, 119
on safety, 225
vendors for, 120
in waiting area, 217
Visibility of location, 43, 67
Vision therapy and sports vision, 103–104
Visiting opthalmogist, 358

W
Waiting, interior, 91–93
Waiting room, main, 85–88
bottlenecks, 86
components of, 87–88
type of seats, 86
Working drawings
alternates to, 281
building permits and, 275
contractor's need for, 274–275
importance, 280–281
Working drawings and schedules process, 274–280
design plan, 275
electrical schedule, 276
elevations, 277–278
finishes and color schedule, 278–279
fixture details and sections, 278
fixture plan, 276–277
graphics, 279–280
mechanical, 280
partition plan, 275–276
reflected ceiling plan, 277
responsibility schedule, 275
signs, exterior and interior, 279